# MORAL ENTANGLEMENTS

# MORAL ENTANGLEMENTS

## The Ancillary-Care Obligations
## of Medical Researchers

Henry S. Richardson

OXFORD
UNIVERSITY PRESS

# OXFORD

## UNIVERSITY PRESS

Oxford University Press is a department of the University of Oxford.
It furthers the University's objective of excellence in research, scholarship,
and education by publishing worldwide.

Oxford    New York
Auckland    Cape Town    Dar es Salaam    Hong Kong    Karachi
Kuala Lumpur    Madrid    Melbourne    Mexico City    Nairobi
New Delhi    Shanghai    Taipei    Toronto

With offices in
Argentina    Austria    Brazil    Chile    Czech Republic    France    Greece
Guatemala    Hungary    Italy    Japan    Poland    Portugal    Singapore
South Korea    Switzerland    Thailand    Turkey    Ukraine    Vietnam

Oxford is a registered trademark of Oxford University Press in the UK
and certain other countries.

Published in the United States of America by
Oxford University Press
198 Madison Avenue, New York, NY 10016

Library of Congress Cataloging-in-Publication Data

Richardson, Henry S.
Moral entanglements : the ancillary-care obligations
of medical researchers / Henry S. Richardson.
p. ; cm.
Includes bibliographical references.
ISBN 978-0-19-538893-0 (alk. paper)
I. Title.
[DNLM: 1. Research Personnel—ethics.    2. Biomedical Research—ethics.
3. Health Care Rationing—ethics.    4. Moral Obligations. W 20.55.E7]

174.2'8—dc23
2012004799

1 3 5 7 9 8 6 4 2
Printed in the United States of America
on acid-free paper

*For Ben and Hope*

# CONTENTS

# LIST OF TABLES, FIGURES, AND CASES

# PREFACE

The issue of medical researchers' ancillary-care obligations to the research participants enrolled in their studies—their obligations to arrange or provide care for their participants that goes beyond what sound science or a study's safety requires—arises pervasively in the trenches. Until the past several years, however, it has been almost entirely ignored by those writing on the ethics of medical research. When Leah Belsky and I published a pair of articles on the topic in 2004, these seem to have been the first writings exclusively focused on the topic. This book sets out a more fully adequate defense and elaboration of the "partial-entrustment model" of researchers' ancillary-care obligations, which we floated in those articles (Belsky & Richardson, 2004; Richardson & Belsky, 2004). In doing so, I am in the uncomfortable position of owning, by default, the received view on an undeservedly obscure issue. The issue remains obscure because, although more has now been written on the topic, not enough of those writing on medical-research ethics have yet taken adequate notice of its practical importance or its theoretical challenges. I own the received view only because, as I write these words, mine is the only fully elaborated view out there. Fortunately, this is now starting to change. In the pages that follow, I engage with several others who have begun to develop alternative positions on ancillary care. I hope above all that the present work stimulates further debate and discussion on the topic and spurs these authors—and others—to articulate competing worked-out views of medical researchers' ancillary-care obligations.

I offer my defense of the partial-entrustment model in the form of a book because no shorter form seemed to me to suffice to set out the necessary arguments. I say this despite having at least dipped my toe into the world of publishing bioethical articles in medical journals, with their bracing insistence on brevity. A number of writers have found the partial-entrustment model appealing or interesting from one angle or another (e.g., Rennie, Sugarman, & the HPTN Ethics Working Group, 2009; Resnik, 2009; Benatar & Singer, 2010; Beskow & Burke, 2010; Cash et al., 2009). Many, I think, find the view intuitively appealing. As a moral philosopher, however, I have felt unsatisfied simply to have a view out there, whether appealing or not. I have sought in recent years to articulate an adequate understanding of what justifies the partial-entrustment model's central claim, namely that when research participants sign up for a medical study via the informed-consent process, they effectively—and without meaning or expecting to—entrust certain limited aspects of their medical needs to the researchers' care. My earlier attempts to do this in article form (e.g., Richardson, 2008a) no longer satisfy me, nor should they satisfy any acute philosophical critic. One of the questions that have always arisen in relation to my earlier attempts to justify the partial-entrustment model's central claim is whether the kind of entrustment it is talking about is peculiar to medical research. From the point of view of reflection on morality and moral principles, it would be odd if this were so. In fact, the more satisfactory justification now set out in Chapter 3 explains ancillary-care obligations in terms of a familiar but theoretically neglected moral phenomenon that crops up in many areas of life, one I call "moral entanglement." Accounting for special ancillary-care obligations on the basis of this idea of moral entanglement provides a satisfactory answer, which my earlier efforts had not, to those (such as Wertheimer, 2011) who are somewhat skeptical of special obligations arising extra-contractually from interactions with others.

From my point of view, it seemed irresponsible to press an ancillary-care view on the public without offering an adequate justification for it. Responding to this need for a justification, however, in relation to a hitherto obscure, if practically urgent, topic of medical-research ethics has generated a challenge for my readers. The good news is that bringing a concern for philosophical rigor together with an attempt to be concrete about the practical challenges that medical researchers face yields some potential illumination in both directions. Moral philosophers have a lot to learn, here—and my own learning process is just a start. Grappling with unfamiliar ancillary-care cases, which arise with myriad variation in medical research, elicits a philosophical specification of principles of special beneficence that is unusually nuanced. Justifying what is an intuitively appealing view on this neglected practical problem by reference to the concept of moral entanglements generates novel insights in moral philosophy about the relation of special obligations to voluntary transactions (the claim will be that ancillary-care obligations are unintended byproducts of voluntary transactions that are undertaken for other purposes). For their part, those with more specialized interests in medical-research ethics—or even medical researchers seeking practical guidance—will see that the philosophical justification offered for the partial-entrustment model helps us in working out the model's recommendations on various practically important matters, such as on the central question of whether participants' ancillary-care claims should be considered waivable (see Chapter 5) and the thorny problems arising in relation to secondary research on samples donated to biobanks (see Chapter 7).

The bad news that corresponds to the way that philosophical analysis and concrete, practical detail inform each other, here, is that various parts of the book may be difficult or dull for one or another type of reader. More practically oriented readers who get through Chapter 2 and find the partial-entrustment model sufficiently appealing or reasonable that they want to proceed straight to its policy implications might skip the philosophical justification offered in Chapter 3 and could even proceed straight to the detailed application of the model, in Chapter 6, to cases in which ancillary care is needed for HIV-AIDS. More philosophical readers, by contrast, will want to concentrate on Chapters 3 through 5 and the first halves of Chapters 7 and 8. Although I feel compelled to offer these suggested shortcuts, I do hope that you will not take me up on them. I hope that the more practically oriented, whether sympathetic to the partial-entrustment model or not, will become puzzled enough about how one might justify medical researchers' ancillary-care obligations that they will want to consider at least one serious effort to do so. And I hope that the more philosophically minded will see how much is to be learned about the very structure of directed duties from grappling with details of the hugely varied ancillary-care cases.

Having voiced my current discomfort, let me express my more overwhelming feeling, which is one of gratitude at my great good fortune in having come across this issue at all, and at having done so in a context ideally suited to facilitate fruitful work on it. This opportunity came about thanks to my having been invited by Ezekiel J. Emanuel to be a Visiting Scholar for the academic year 2002–3 at the Department of Clinical Bioethics (now simply known as the Department of Bioethics) at the National Institutes of Health in Bethesda, Maryland, U.S.A. Not having done previous work in the ethics of medical research, I accepted this generous invitation thinking that I would attempt to discover some needed epicycle in our theoretical accounts of the morality of medical research enrolling children as subjects. Although this remains a topic of fascination to me, it rather quickly became clear that I was not going to be a person who would make any great headway on that topic. To the best of my recollection, the ancillary-care issue arose in conversations with Christine Grady and David Wendler, each members of the department's faculty. Grady had been grappling with the unfamiliar issue in internal NIH discussions of what to do about participants in HIV vaccine trials who become HIV positive (as such trials anticipate that some will). Wendler had given a pioneering presentation on the ethics of ancillary care at a research-ethics workshop run by the department in Kampala, Uganda, in March 2002. Zeke Emanuel was soon in on our discussions, and we decided that this would be a fine topic for me to spend some months on. (As the elapsed time indicates, the work has expanded beyond that. The NIH department even had me back, as a half-time Visiting Scholar for 2006, to work more on the issue.) In my initial work on the subject, I was lucky to be paired with Leah Belsky, one of the department's outstanding group of post-baccalaureate fellows. Sustained and stretched by the department's remarkable commitment to "combative collegiality," Belsky and I sat together and worked line-by-line on umpteen drafts (up through version 59H) of our first ancillary-care article, sharing ideas about everything from moral principles to hyphens (yes when "ancillary care" is used as an adjective; no otherwise, we decided). In the intervening years, Belsky has completed a degree at Yale Law School and moved on to tackling other important issues. I hope she remembers our collaboration with at least a smidge of the fondness with which I do. Her compassionate sense of the need that many have for ancillary care, her analytic acuity, and her philosophical imagination were great assets in our work together.

As is obvious, then, I owe a debt of gratitude first and foremost to Zeke Emanuel, Christine Grady, David Wendler, and the whole NIH Bioethics Department—including several cohorts of fellows, post-baccalaureate and post-doctoral—who continued to provide invaluable support and feedback as I kept working on this issue. (I exempt Belsky from such thanks: we were in it together.) Three other faculty members of the department, though perhaps not part of my very first conversations on the subject, offered support and constructively critical comments from very early on: Reidar Lie, Franklin G. Miller, and Alan Wertheimer. I am lucky indeed to have gained an education in research ethics from them and from all of the department's faculty. Furthermore, because the department is housed in NIH's Clinical Center, it provides an ideal base for coming to have some concrete sense of how medical research proceeds. Many in the Clinical Center were helpful to Belsky and me. I am particularly grateful to have been allowed to go on teaching rounds with Drs. Stephen Chanock and Steven Holland, to speak with members of the Parasitology and International Programs Branch of the National Institute of Allergy and Infectious Diseases, led by Dr. Lee Hall, and to learn about the ancillary-care issues related to mental health from Dr. Donald Rosenstein. Each of these researchers also provided feedback on our early ancillary-care work. NIH's Clinical Center being a rather rarefied and not fully typical research environment, I am also grateful to have had a chance—again thanks to Zeke Emanuel, Reidar Lie, and the Department of Bioethics—to participate in two seminars on medical-research ethics in Africa, where I was able to discuss ancillary-care issues with groups of African researchers: the 3rd Africa Conference on Ethical Aspects of Clinical Research in Developing Countries in Kampala, Uganda, in March 2003, and the Advanced Workshop on Research Ethics in Kiwengwa, Tanzania, in December 2004.

As I have continued to work on ancillary-care issues, I have benefited from the advice, encouragement, knowledge, and constructive criticism of a great many people—far too many, I am afraid, to list here. Many of these people are listed in the acknowledgments of my articles on ancillary care. Here I would like to reiterate this thanks. A few, however, I must single out. Frank Miller and Dave Wendler have continued to offer pointed and helpful comments. From the beginning of my work with Belsky down through my latest draft, Leif Wenar, in voluminous email correspondence, has provided important and challenging feedback. Wenar's "least-cost threat avoider view," which I discuss in Chapter 3 and which he had developed in the context of debates about global justice, could well serve as a basis for a worthy rival to the partial-entrustment model. Having this potential rival view constantly in mind as I have been developing my own has, I feel, helped keep me honest and humble in my own claims. Crucial encouragement to work out and articulate an adequate philosophical justification of the partial-entrustment model came from David Copp, who also provided incisive comments on the paper that is the basis of Chapter 3. More recently, as I have been working both on those justificatory arguments and on various practical implications of the model, I have benefited hugely from Maria Merritt's general insights and detailed comments on many of the chapters, which were informed and enriched by her own developing views on ancillary-care obligations. I learned much presenting the view at King's College London, particularly from the reactions of Neema Sofaer and Carwyn Hooper. I also presented the view at the Global Health Seminar at Yale, where I gained much from the participants and from its leaders, Thomas Pogge and Jennifer Prah Ruger, and at the Bioethics Workshop at New York University, where Matthew Liao's questioning was particularly helpful.

The Workshop on the Ancillary-Care Obligations of Medical Researchers Working in Developing Countries, which I organized at Georgetown in October 2006, helped convince me that this issue urgently needs to be explicitly addressed by the medical-research community. I learned a tremendous amount from my fellow presenters, who included medical researchers from the United States and Africa, bioethicists, government officials, and pharmaceutical-company executives. I learned even more from the process of writing a paper stating the consensus of the group (Participants, 2008), on which I worked with Christine Grady and Reidar Lie. I am grateful for the forthrightness and reasonableness of all fourteen of my co-authors, whose names are listed in the article and in note 9 in Chapter 8. To Alexander Capron, the one workshop presenter who was too busy or too wise to get involved in the cumbersome process of producing the consensus paper, I owe a debt of a different kind. It was he who gave me my start with bioethics—and specifically with the privacy issues that are central in Chapter 3—in the summer of 1981, when I was an intern at the President's Commission for the Study of Ethical Problems in Medicine and Biomedical and Behavioral Research, where he was the Executive Director.

If the first year I spent at NIH's Department of Bioethics enabled me to get going on the ancillary-care issue and my return visit there enabled me to begin deepening my view, the completion of this book has been made possible by some more recent research support. I am grateful to Georgetown University for a Senior Faculty Fellowship and to the National Endowment for the Humanities for a Fellowship for University Teachers (FA-53986-08) supporting the research leave in 2008–9 that ultimately made it possible for me to write this book.

# Chapter 1

# Medical Researchers' Ancillary-Care Obligations: A Neglected Issue

A medical researcher may be interested in transmission of malaria across the placenta. To study this, she may have recruited a group of pregnant malaria sufferers in rural West Africa into an observational study of pregnant women and their babies. Although pursuing a narrow and well-defined study objective having to do with malaria, it is inevitable that, in working with her human research participants in this population, she will encounter in them various other diseases and conditions that are threatening to their health but unrelated to malaria. It is likely that, aside from access to the research team's clinic, the participants have little access to modern medicine. Inevitably, then, the question will arise: Should this malaria researcher devote some of the team's budgetary and personnel resources to treating these other conditions, insofar as they are able, or to helping their participants get treatment elsewhere? This is a difficult moral question, and one on which this researcher would benefit from guidance. Analogues of this question arise in all kinds of medical research involving human subjects. To date, however, no authoritative ethical guidance on this sort of issue is available. This book aims to contribute towards the formulation of such guidance by articulating and defending a view about how to answer such questions.

The view defended here holds that this malaria researcher does have ancillary-care obligations regarding some of these other conditions found in the subjects. More generally, according to the view I defend—the "partial-entrustment model" of medical researchers' ancillary-care obligations—medical researchers have a special obligation to help their research participants with medical needs that come to light via the carrying out of study procedures, subject to the research participants' claims for such care surviving a contextualized test of their "strength."

The ancillary-care question for medical researchers, most generally, is what medical researchers should do when—as foreseen or by surprise—they encounter in one of their study participants an urgent or important medical need that arises from a disease or condition other than the one the researchers are studying. Although a complex regulatory apparatus and a correspondingly detailed critical literature has grown up around the ethics of medical research over the past few decades, these have almost entirely ignored the question of medical researchers' ancillary-care obligations. For completely understandable historical reasons, these are almost entirely focused on two aims: avoiding exploiting research participants and avoiding exposing them to unnecessary or excessive risks. Established procedures of obtaining participants' informed consent and subjecting all proposed trials involving human subjects to review by Institutional Review Boards (IRBs) or Research Ethics Committees (RECs) serve these goals reasonably well. The guidelines and literature pertaining to medical research ethics have, however, largely tended to ignore researchers' specific duties of beneficence towards participants. In particular, they have ignored the possibility of ancillary-care duties arising in the context of medical research.

In the context of medical research, we may think of "ancillary care" as medical care that the research subjects need but that is not required to make a study scientifically valid, to ensure a study's safety, or to redress research injuries.[1] This definition is crafted so as to keep our attention focused on instances where the grounds for providing care that is otherwise not "research related" have to do with the promotion of the participants' health or well-being, instead of stemming from the research aims of the scientists or from the imperative not to harm participants. Thus, providing medical care is sometimes built into the study design. Beyond that, general duties of non-maleficence may make medical care for trial participants morally necessary—either because it is wrong to expose people to medical risk in pursuit of a scientifically insignificant question (an issue of sound science) or because it is wrong to expose people to undue medical risk, period (an issue of safety). Such issues came to the fore, with special attention to developing countries, at the end of the last century (e.g., Angell, 1997; Lurie & Wolf, 1997; Varmus & Satcher, 1997; Crouch & Arras, 1998), in debates about the "standard of care" for the disease or condition under study that should be guaranteed to all study participants, including those in the control arm. In addition, if participation in research ends up harming the participants, then the researchers may well owe some care to the participants by way of compensation. But researchers will also discover in their subjects diseases and other medical problems that are *not* what is under study—diseases and conditions that the researchers did not cause but that call for care and treatment that have no part in the scientific protocol they are pursuing. These other problems are not covered in the same way by the issues of safety and sound science. Do the researchers have a responsibility to provide medical care for those problems? Do the research participants have any moral claim on the researchers for ancillary care? To

---

1. The definition in the text is essentially that given in Belsky & Richardson (2004): 1494–1496.

speak of "ancillary care," then, is emphatically not to speak of care that is unimportant or as beyond the responsibilities of researchers' role—a meaning that some might glean from the term "ancillary" (cf. Cash et al., 2009, 109)—but to focus on the neglected question of whether medical researchers have duties of care that arise from grounds other than the well-understood ones of sound science and safety.

Ancillary-care needs can arise in very different ways and in very different contexts. Consider first the following simplified case, again involving malaria, but this time specifying how the ancillary-care need is discovered:

> *Malaria Researchers and Schistosomiasis:* In certain parts of Africa, both malaria and schistosomiasis—each a dangerous and debilitating parasitic disease—are endemic. Malaria researchers working in those areas will often confirm malaria diagnoses by checking fluid samples under the microscope. When they do so, they are likely to see, and so to diagnose infection by, the schistosomiasis parasite as well. Do they owe the participants care for their schistosomiasis? We may realistically suppose that, in many of the areas where such research is carried out, if the participants do not receive this medical care from the researchers, they will not receive it at all.[2]

Nor are significant questions about medical researchers' ancillary-care obligations confined to developing-country settings. The

---

2. One disadvantage of this example is that while it is relatively easy temporarily to reduce the number of schistosomiasis parasites infecting an individual, doing this has a fairly marginal long-term impact on this individual's health, given the likelihood that an infected individual will be reinfected because of poor sanitation or poor access to clean water. Ancillary-care issues can arise in many other combinations: finding HIV in malaria trial, finding heart defects in a tuberculosis trial, etc. I retain the Malaria and Schistosomiasis example because it has entered the research-ethics literature in a modest way.

following case illustrates how they can arise largely independently of overall resource constraints:

> *Brain Scans:* In university medical centers and other advanced research labs, it has become quite popular to conduct brain scans of normal volunteers to see what their brains look like when they are thinking about partisan politics or about the trolley problem. One study has shown that a diagnostic reading of these scans would result in 1% of these "normals" being referred to a clinician for urgent follow-up (Katzman, Dagher, & Patronas, 1999; cf. Illes et al., 2006). Should the researchers read the scans diagnostically? (Or, better, to help avoid false positives, should they order a physician-read diagnostic-quality scan for every normal volunteer they enroll in a brain-scan study?)

In the malaria example, the subjects are poor and, presumably, lacking any medical insurance. In the Brain Scans case, the subjects may well be neither poor nor uninsured. Even so, there may remain non-trivial ancillary ways that the researchers might be uniquely able to provide them with the help that they need.

As these contrasting illustrations indicate, ancillary-care needs arise pervasively, and in very different ways, in the context of medical research. Fortunately, although the issue had been almost entirely neglected both by research-ethics guidelines and by the literature on medical research ethics, attention is now being paid. It will be illuminating to look at one concrete problem that brought the issue to people's attention.

## A PERPLEXING ISSUE

As far as I know, this issue of medical researchers' ancillary-care obligations first forced itself onto the awareness of policymakers and specialists in medical research ethics in the context of the large HIV-vaccine trials in developing countries that began being conducted and planned at the turn of the last century. Because the HIV virus presents itself in different variants (different clades) in different parts of the world, and because developing countries disproportionately suffer the ravages of HIV-AIDS, it has been imperative to try to develop vaccines effective against the forms of HIV prevalent there. Officials anticipating large, randomized controlled effectiveness trials of HIV vaccine in developing countries could foresee the following heartbreaking scenario: Trials of a new vaccine's effectiveness necessarily involve large numbers of participants. Generally, the aim is to find a population that is somewhat at risk and to use randomization between the trial vaccine and placebo to see if there is a difference in the infection rate. This means that it will involve a significant number of participants whom the researchers will find to be HIV positive. One three-year trial of a regimen of two trial vaccines for HIV, begun in Thailand in 2006 as a collaboration between the U.S. military and the Thai government, involved 16,402 volunteer subjects. One hundred twenty-five of these became HIV positive during the course of the trial (McNeil, Jr., 2009; cf. Rerks-Ngarm et al., 2009). As I write this, scientists are still debating whether the difference between the number of those who became infected from the placebo arm of the trial (74) and the number from the active arm (51) represents a significant level of effectiveness. What is beyond question, however, is that the trial vaccines did not biologically cause these 125 people to become HIV positive. These vaccines do not involve an ingredient even remotely close to a live vaccine. It is possible that mere participation in such a trial might induce a false sense of security in some participants, leading them to riskier sexual behavior; but HIV researchers have learned to be careful to protect against this danger with thorough counseling. Further, one recent interview study in

South Africa found considerable acceptance of the idea that, given this kind of warning, it is the participants' responsibility to engage in safe sex. As a young patient from a rural primary-care clinic in KwaZulu Natal put it, "[i]t is not the researchers' fault they [the participants] were careless because they were told to use protection" (Barsdorf et al., 2010, 83).

Once participants in a vaccine trial become HIV positive, or relatively soon thereafter, their participation in the trial—as dictated by the trial's "protocol," its official design document—ended. Since the Thai trial also assessed the viral load of those infected, it continued to work with them for the full three years of the trial, independently of when they became infected. Any subsequent care for these people's HIV infection would count as ancillary care.

Thailand's policies make the antiretroviral drugs needed for effective HIV care relatively widely and cheaply available. By contrast, when officials early in this century were contemplating such large-scale HIV-vaccine trials in developing countries, in Africa as well as in Southeast Asia, antiretrovirals were much more expensive and government policies for making them available to those who need them were much less well developed. Accordingly, these officials came face-to-face with the unpleasant fact that HIV-vaccine trials could be expected to bring to light urgent needs for life-saving medicines that would be hideously expensive to provide. This quandary did much to bring the issue of medical researchers' ancillary-care obligations to consciousness.[3] On March 16, 2005, the National Institutes of Health, the U.S. government's body that conducts and funds a vast amount of medical research, issued a guidance memorandum on the related issue of

3. Edmund Pincoffs (1971) influentially made the point that it is a mistake to orient ethical theory entirely towards quandaries. Compatibly with the soundness of that point, however, we must recognize that quandaries have their importance.

post-trial provision of antiretrovirals to participants in trials of those drugs (NIH, 2005):

> The NIH's authority to "encourage and support research" does not extend to providing treatment following the completion of that research. 42 USC 284(b)(1)(A). It is important that trial participants who receive antiretroviral treatment in NIH-supported/funded antiretroviral treatment trials have the option to continue to receive antiretroviral treatment following their completion of the trial. Thus, the NIH recommends NIH-supported/funded investigators engage in a dialogue with host countries' authorities and other stakeholders in order to facilitate the inclusion of these populations in available in-country antiretroviral treatment programs and when applications are made for treatment programs through outside agencies.

While the realities that underlay this stance have continued to shift, it is important to recognize the reality of the tensions expressed here (cf. MacQueen et al., 2008, 15). The NIH officials were caught between dire human needs of individual research participants, which they sought to identify some way of meeting, and their responsibility to support medical research for the long-term benefit of humankind.

Tension between promoting long-term scientific objectives and the needs of individual research participants might take many forms (cf. Merritt, 2005). For instance, it might take the form of a conflict between clinical reasons to tailor drug dosages to individual variations in response and a drug trial's need for uniformity. A central aim of the present book is to elaborate a principled framework for addressing this general tension as it arises in clashes between the ancillary-care needs of individual research participants and the promotion of long-term scientific objectives. I have two general reasons for sticking to this version of the tension. First, the issue of medical researchers' ancillary-care obligations has been woefully neglected. Second, the principled basis for addressing the tension that I have to offer is relevant only to ancillary-care obligations.

A principled framework is needed so that ancillary-care decisions are not left merely to ad hoc pressure politics or idiosyncratic intuition. Furthermore, as I shall argue, there are important principles that bear on these decisions, indicating lines along which a principled solution can be constructed. Amazingly for any moral issue, and in particular for one in the area of medical research ethics, this construction must proceed largely from scratch. In 2004, my colleague Leah Belsky and I published a pair of articles on ancillary care (Belsky & Richardson, 2004; Richardson & Belsky, 2004). At that time, there was almost nothing on the issue in the published literature.[4] Relatedly—I think because of the way in which the medical research ethics establishment grew up in response to terrible cases of abuse—there is currently no settled set of expectations or guidelines about medical researchers' ancillary-care obligations in such cases (cf. Participants, 2008). Indeed, there are very few data about what medical researchers do in such cases or think they ought to do, and correspondingly little shared understanding about these important practical matters.[5]

Further, that medical researchers have ancillary-care obligations is not simply obvious, nor can a clear position on this issue be simply read off of existing understandings of medical researchers' professional obligations. In fact, the general tension that makes the issue of ancillary care a difficult one in contexts such as HIV-vaccine trials is aligned around a fault line at the heart of con-

---

4. The issue had been touched upon by the Nuffield Council on Bioethics (2002, 97).
5. Chapter 7 will go over this fact in more detail, mentioning the studies of which I am aware.

temporary understandings of medical researchers' roles. Although teams of medical researchers are often large and diverse, the principal investigators are usually physicians who naturally take their orientation from a physician's emphasis on care for patients. Yet as research scientists, they also understandably sense—and indeed rightfully acknowledge—an allegiance to their scientific mission. Specialists in medical research ethics have been debating for years whether it is a mistake to assimilate medical researchers' obligations to those of physicians. In this general debate, my sense is that the side that has been emphasizing the morally *sui generis* features of medical research has recently had the upper hand (see, e.g., Miller & Rosenstein, 2003). Even if that is not the correct view, however, the fact remains that the doubts and uncertainties about how to characterize the profession of medical research bear upon exactly the kind of tension that appears at the nub of many ancillary-care questions, making recourse to existing understandings of medical researchers' professional roles quite treacherous.

These doubts and tensions also affect the ways individual medical researchers respond when issues of ancillary care are raised. I have found that medical researchers faced with the issue commonly voice one of two polar reactions to the question of whether medical researchers have special ancillary-care obligations, reactions that reflect the ambiguity of the role of the medical researcher, poised as it is between science and medicine. A common first reaction among physicians who are medical researchers is to affirm a very broad commitment to ancillary-care responsibilities, on the basis not of any particular account about how these arise but instead of an assimilation of researchers' duties towards their subjects to physicians' duties towards their patients. On this view, researchers have a duty to promote the subjects' health in all ways the researchers are competent to, whether by providing the care themselves, organizing it, or referring the subjects to an appropriate specialist.

After more probing, however, second thoughts arise. When faced with cases such as Malaria Researchers and Schistosomiasis or that of HIV-vaccine trials, researchers soon realize that, in "resource-poor" settings, at least, this assimilation of researchers' duties to physicians' would often entail a significant diversion of resources away from their research efforts. In response, the second common reaction arises, which is to deny that researchers, who are scientists first and foremost, have any special ancillary-care obligations.[6] Not unless they have expressly agreed to them, that is, in an essentially contractual exchange of promises occurring when the subjects are enrolled in a trial. Some will one-sidedly locate a deeper rationale for resisting special ancillary-care responsibilities in their commitment to the scientific *telos* of medical research—namely, contributing to general knowledge pertinent to human health. This second common reaction has two variants. An extreme variant holds that providing ancillary care to research subjects is *permissible* only if offering it is necessary to recruit an adequate number of subjects for the trial in question—and then only when the scientific benefits of recruiting subjects outweigh the scientific opportunity costs of using those resources otherwise. When such conditions are met, providing ancillary care can be seen as contributing to the aims of science. A weaker variant of this second common reaction would leave more leeway for researchers to promise ancillary care at their discretion, but still insist that none is owed unless it has been promised.

Neither of these polar reactions presents a morally acceptable response. Casting medical researchers as narrowly focused scientists who lack ancillary-care obligations takes too little account of how they crucially interact with the human subjects of their

6. These two responses illustrate what Barbara Herman identifies as "two independent currents in our moral understanding," moral responsiveness to faced need and moral protection of agential prerogative (Herman, 2001, 228).

research. Assimilating medical researchers to clinical physicians, by contrast, takes too little account of their responsibilities to promote the advancement of science, threatening to overwhelm their research activities with ancillary duties. Now that some attention is being paid to the question of medical researchers' ancillary-care obligations, there seems to be an emerging consensus in favor of the view that there are some such special duties of care, but that they are limited, and do not extend to all of a study participants' health needs (e.g., Miller, Mello, & Joffe, 2008; Participants, 2008; Barsdorf et al., 2010). My task here, again, is to spell out and defend a principled basis for such an intermediate position.

## ANCILLARY-CARE OBLIGATIONS AND THE DISTINCTIVE ANCILLARY-CARE OBLIGATION

Part of the awkwardness of defending what has become, merely by default, the leading view on the question of ancillary care is that the articles that Belsky and I published in 2004 framed the nascent discussions on the issue using terminology that was less than ideal. The terminology was, in one respect, an unconscious byproduct of our aims. Our work sought both to articulate this long-neglected question and to identify a core ancillary-care obligation specific to the researcher–participant relationship. That is, we aimed both to call attention to the *issue* of medical researchers' ancillary-care obligations and to articulate a specific *account* of the distinctive basis of such obligations. We used the phrase "ancillary-care obligations" both to label the issue and to label the account. This dual usage has already led to some confusion. The reason is simple: there are many possible moral grounds for medical researchers having, in any given situation, some obligation to provide ancillary care. Important among these are grounds of *gratitude* (if the research participants have willingly undergone considerable inconvenience and discomfort for the sake of science) and grounds of being relatively uniquely situated to respond easily to dire need, grounds that philosophers think of as falling under the heading of the principle of *rescue* (McIntyre, 1994; Scanlon, 1998). (What if the researchers *promised* participants care in order to recruit them into the trial? Definitionally—at least if these promises were needed in order to recruit an adequate number of participants—this would arguably not count as "ancillary care," as defined above, for the care involved would count as a part of the study's scientific design.)[7] These grounds of gratitude and rescue are not specific to the researcher–participant relationship. Yet Belsky and I also maintained that—compatibly with the existence of these more general grounds for providing ancillary care in some cases, there is also a distinctive set of grounds for ancillary-care obligations that is specific to the researcher–participant relationship. These latter grounds, we rather confusingly maintained, make up the core of medical researchers' ancillary-care obligations, and yield obligations of limited scope.

I still think our view was sound. To set it out more clearly, however, we must now distinguish:

- *the issue* of when medical researchers are obligated to provide ancillary care

7. The first definition of "ancillary care" that Belsky and I offered (for the context of medical research) was as follows: "care not required by sound science, safe trial conduct, morally optional promises, or redressing subject injury" (Richardson & Belsky, 2004, 26). On that definition, it is analytic that care required solely by a prior promise is not "ancillary care." Our subsequent definition, in a later paper that same year (quoted in the text above, at n. 1), which is the one I will continue to use here, dropped this mention of promises. Our thought was that as researchers become enlightened as to their ancillary-care obligations, this might lead them to make a habit of promising to provide reasonable ancillary care. If they did so, that surely would not erase their ancillary-care obligations, but rather reinforce them with a promise (which, though it pertains to morally obligatory actions, is nonetheless, as a promise, morally optional).

and

- *the moral grounds* on the basis of which medical researchers are obligated, in given circumstances, to provide ancillary care

from

- *the distinctive ancillary-care obligation* (if any) that arises in the context of the relationship between medical researchers and their research participants and explains why the researchers are specially obligated to those participants in particular.

While meaning to cover the issue quite comprehensively and not intending to leave out any important potential moral grounds for ancillary-care obligations, my principal aim in this book is to explain the distinctive ancillary-care obligation that binds a particular set of researchers to the participants in their studies. In doing so, however, I do not claim that this distinctive ancillary-care obligation exhausts the potential moral grounds why, in given circumstances, medical researchers ought to provide ancillary care (Table 1).

The claim that there is such a distinctive ancillary-care obligation is a controversial one that will need defense. Within the reasonable range of views that is marked out by rejecting the two polar reactions to the question of ancillary care, it would be quite possible to stake out a position that did without, or even denied the existence of, any such distinctive obligation. One might, for instance, appeal to Robert Goodin (1985), the very general thesis of which was that we each have a duty to protect the vulnerable. Alternatively, one might extend Leif Wenar's notion of a "least-cost threat avoider," which he developed to account for duties towards the severely deprived (Wenar, 2007; cf. Miller, 2001). The general thought would be that research subjects who need ancillary care are quite vulnerable to significant losses of well-being, or even of

Table 1  GENERAL AND SPECIAL GROUNDS
OF ANCILLARY-CARE OBLIGATIONS

| MEDICAL RESEARCHERS' ANCILLARY-CARE OBLIGATIONS | |
| --- | --- |
| **THE ISSUE THEREOF** | |
| When are medical researchers obligated to provide ancillary care? | |
| **GROUNDS THEREFOR** | |
| A. *General Grounds* | B. *Special Grounds* |
| – Rescue | – Gratitude |
| – Justice | – Promises |
| – Etc. | – The distinctive ancillary-care obligation |

life, and that the medical researchers are, in the relevant respects, best positioned to help them relatively easily. In contrast to either of these sorts of view, which allocate duties of aid on an impartial basis, and which I will discuss in Chapter 3, the view I seek to defend attributes intrinsic moral importance to the relationship between researchers and research participants—a relationship that has arisen from particular (although generally characterizable) transactions between them.

Putting this point together with the previous one, one can see that it is perfectly coherent to recognize both general and special grounds for ancillary-care claims. Attributing intrinsic moral importance to the relationship between researchers and participants, as a basis of a distinctive moral obligation that the former owe the latter, is compatible with *also* recognizing the moral importance of general moral duties such as the duty of rescue (Hawkins, 2006).[8] And, in fact, as has been emphasized by Merritt, Taylor, and Mullany (2010), it should be obvious that some ancillary care is owed to research subjects simply on the basis of the duty of rescue. If a participant has a heart attack while visiting the research clinic, researchers owe it to him or her to do what they can to stabilize things and mitigate the heart attack's ill effects. Since schistosomiasis is a parasitical infection that can be at least temporarily relieved by administering anti-helminthic drugs that cost pennies a dose, the researchers in Malaria Researchers and Schistosomiasis should clearly make these drugs available for this ancillary care if they have them handy. In each of these cases, since easy, low-cost steps can make a huge difference to individuals' health and well-being, and since the researchers are in a relatively unique position to provide this easy help, the duty of rescue supports their doing so.

A distinctive ancillary-care obligation, however, starts to come into view once one gets outside of cases covered by the duty of rescue. As an obligation tied to the relationship between researchers and their research participants, this distinctive obligation departs from impartiality in two directions at once. First, it singles out the researchers, and the research team more broadly,[9] as having special obligations that go beyond anything implied by impartial duties. I think that this implication is at least plausible. To test it first with regard to relatively easily provided ancillary care: Suppose that in the rural area where the malaria researchers

8. Some philosophers have sharply distinguished natural duties, incumbent on people independently of any voluntary choice or transaction, from obligations, which do arise from voluntary choices or transactions. While I do not mean to endorse this strict dichotomy, I do find it natural to use the terms "obligation" and "duty" in ways that at least chime in with a rough contrast along these lines.

9. See Chapter 7 for a discussion of the complexities introduced by the fact that research teams typically involve many different sorts of collaborating specialists working with the support of a number of different funding and sponsoring institutions.

of Malaria Researchers and Schistosomiasis are operating there is also another medical study going on, one conducted by schistosomiasis specialists. This might well mean that, even though the malaria researchers could alleviate the schistosomiasis they find in their participants relatively easily, the schistosomiasis researchers in the next village could do so even more easily. Impartially, an approach such as the least-cost threat avoider approach might suggest that the malaria-study participant ought to go to the schistosomiasis researchers for schistosomiasis care, even if this individual is not a participant in the schistosomiasis study.[10] The distinctive ancillary-care obligation might well imply, however, that the chief moral obligation nonetheless rests on the shoulders of the malaria researchers, whose study participants we are talking about. One rather crude way to bring out this point would be to ask—as we ultimately must, in the end of the day—who is to pay for the drugs and the care in question. Even if it is efficient and workable to refer these individuals to the schistosomiasis researchers in the next village for their schistosomiasis care—and that is an important "if"—there remains the independent question of whose budget should get charged for the personnel time and the schistosomiasis drugs used. A distinctive ancillary-care obligation would provide a basis for arguing that these budgetary burdens should be borne by the malaria researchers, whose participants are the ones who need such care.[11] (We are supposing that such care is not otherwise available in the locality on a free, public basis.)

10. There would be some transactional cost, of course, in this individual's striking up a relationship with a new set of doctors; but for present purposes we can suppose that administering schistosomiasis care would be so much easier for the schistosomiasis researchers that the "cost" of care remains less if they provide it.
11. In this book, I concentrate on laying out the principled basis for making such an argument, rather than on the more complex issue of how competing moral arguments bear on what, all things considered, we ought to do. I am grateful to Maria Merritt for pressing me on this question.

What does it mean for the researchers to bear a special responsibility of this sort, one that persists despite not being supported by impartial considerations? This can be seen in cases where providing the ancillary care is not easy at all. Consider the following case, which is based on a real case that arose during a community-based HIV-AIDS study in western Uganda:

*Advanced Cervical Cancer in a HIV-transmission Study:* A substudy in a long-term community-based study of HIV transmission rates in western Uganda considered the effect of other sexually transmitted diseases (STDs) on the rate of HIV transmission. The presence of other STDs was confirmed and tracked by means of physical exams at the community clinics that had been set up as part of the longer-term research effort. In one of these exams, one of the participating women was found to have advanced and life-threatening cervical cancer. Saving her life would have required relatively complex surgery. After carefully looking into all of the options, the researchers at the clinic determined that the needed surgery was not available in Uganda, and that the woman would have to be flown to Kenya for it. With regret, they decided that they could not afford to fly her to Kenya for the surgery.

Clearly, this case is a tragic one. At present, I do not mean to debate whether or not the researchers made the right choice.[12] Rather, I want to draw your attention to part of what makes this a particularly tragic situation. If there is a distinctive ancillary-care obligation, these feelings reflected a genuine moral responsibility.

12. See Richardson (2008a, 265) for discussion of another tragic case, involving researchers conducting a trial in Benin of vaginal microbicides who discovered a life-threatening ectopic pregnancy that would, like the cervical cancer discovered in Uganda, have required surgery in a neighboring country.

If there is a distinctive ancillary-care obligation, it would, in addition to picking out researchers for special obligations, also pick out their study participants for special claims. Looking at things from the side of those who need care, different aspects of an impartial approach come into view. Where medical resources are scarce—in short, in some sense, everywhere—we often have reason to think about impartial grounds for allocating them. Scarce vaccines, for instance, should go to those most at risk or perhaps to those whose chance at "fair innings" in life is most at risk.[13] In coping with the HIV-AIDS pandemic, governments have struggled to come up with defensible systems for fairly allocating a limited stock of antiretroviral medication—along with the limited set of trained personnel needed to administer it. Consider such a country, and suppose now that U.S. or European sponsors fund a large HIV-vaccine trial there. If there is a distinctive ancillary-care obligation, then these vaccine researchers may well have an ancillary-care duty to see to it that those of their participants who are found to be HIV positive during the course of the trial receive antiretroviral treatment. If need be, these researchers, or their institutional sponsors, could pay for this treatment. Even so, this would be to give these research participants priority over other HIV-positive people in that country who have been waiting for such treatment. From an impartial point of view, that might seem unjust or unfair (cf. Merritt & Grady, 2006). Without denying that, however, and without insisting that ancillary-care considerations always override impartial justice or fairness, the defender of a distinctive ancillary-care obligation will hold that such an obligation can provide a justified basis for departing from impartiality in such cases. That is because this distinctive obligation gives rise to a special claim, a claim that a research participant has on those researchers who are conducting the trial in which he or she is participating.

13. For a variant of the latter, "fair innings" idea, see Emanuel & Wertheimer (2006).

A distinctive ancillary-care obligation thus would reflect something about the relationship between medical researchers and research participants. This would be so even if this distinctive obligation supplements, rather than supplanting, some general obligations, such as the duty of rescue, that also ground ancillary-care obligations. But what is it about the relationship between medical researchers and research participants that might be morally relevant and might explain such special obligations, with the corresponding claims? It cannot be the mere fact of a "relationship." Human relationships are tremendously varied. Researchers may have a relationship with the bartender and waitresses at the bar where they regularly go on Friday evening, learning their names and engaging in friendly banter with them; but this relationship is presumably not the sort on which any significant and distinctive ancillary-care obligation might rest.

One line of criticism of the account of medical researchers' ancillary-care obligations that Belsky and I offered has been that, in being focused (in a way that I will explain) on what emerges from carrying out study procedures, it is too limited in scope (Dickert et al., 2007; Dickert & Wendler, 2009a). It leaves out, for instance, diseases or conditions that are apparent to the naked eye (or at least, to the naked eye of a trained person). However, if a distinctive ancillary-care obligation is to be grounded in the relationship between researchers and their research participants, some such limitation of scope is to be expected. Intuitively, just as their informal relationships with the wait staff at the local bar or the hospital janitor will not ground medical researchers' distinctive ancillary-care obligations, so, too, will their informal interactions with people who happen also to be their research participants be irrelevant to any such distinctive obligation. If a researcher happens upon one of her research participants at the local bar on a Friday night and something transpires there—if the participant's tank top reveals a worrisome-looking skin lesion that the researcher had not seen before or if the participant suddenly starts having a heart attack in the bar—it may very well be that the researcher, especially in light of her medical training, has a rescue-based obligation to intervene in some way. It does not seem plausible to say, however, that the researcher additionally has a special obligation, somehow grounded in her status as a researcher who has enrolled this individual as a research participant, to do something about this lesion or this heart attack.[14] Any distinctive ancillary-care obligation specially grounded in this relationship may be expected, in other words, to follow in some ways the contours of the core interactions around which the relationship is defined.[15]

14. On the basis of considerations that will emerge with the two variants of the case of the Massage Therapist and the Mole, to be discussed in Chapter 3, the partial-entrustment model of researchers' special ancillary-care obligations, which I defend, would maintain this moral differentiation—that is, the one between (a) information surfacing as a result of nonprofessional interactions between researchers and their study participants and (b) information surfacing as a result of carrying out study procedures—even for cases in which the information is topically within the scope of the research (so, even if the lesion is seen in the bar by a dermatology researcher or the incipient heart attack is observed in the bar by a cardiology researcher). I am grateful to Dave Wendler for pressing me to clarify this point.
15. I do not mean to claim that this scope limitation holds of all special relationships. In particular, if the special relationship arises from one's having harmed someone in some way, one may end up owing quite an unrestricted duty of care, by way of making amends, as a result.

# Chapter 2

# Special Ancillary-Care Obligations: The Partial-Entrustment Model

We have seen that medical researchers' ancillary-care obligations seem to involve a special moral relationship between researchers and their research participants, such that the researchers have some special obligation to provide and facilitate ancillary care that participants in their studies need, at least in some circumstances. But what is the nature of this special obligation, what are its limits, and how should we think about the variations in circumstance that might be relevant to determining how far these obligations extend? In this chapter, I lay out the basic position on this that this book will defend and elaborate. It is the position that I first set out in a pair of articles with Leah Belsky (Belsky & Richardson, 2004; Richardson & Belsky, 2004).[1] Because we gave a central role, in setting out the position, to the idea that the participants effectively entrust some (but not all) aspects of their health to the researchers, this position has become known as the "partial-entrustment view." While the following chapter, which will delve more deeply into the philosophical basis for the view, will provide alternative ways of thinking about it, it will also support seeing the distinctive ancillary-care obligation in terms of entrustment. Accordingly,

---

1. The present chapter draws heavily on these two articles, while updating the presentation and revising the ideas in various respects.

I will retain this label, and will seek to explain in this chapter the special sense in which entrustment is involved.

According to the partial-entrustment account, the special ancillary-care obligation is both limited in scope and hedged in relation to various circumstantial factors that, together, affect the "strength" of the obligation. The core task of the present chapter is to set out this two-part account.

## THE EXISTING LACK OF GUIDANCE

We have seen that the issue of ancillary care illustrates the way in which the profession of medical research sits poised awkwardly and somewhat unstably between two other professions, the goals of which are simpler and the ethics of which are more settled: those of the physician and the scientist. Sometimes—as when a physician has enrolled one of her patients in a drug trial and the dosage prescribed by the trial seems not fully to suit her patient, or when a study of genetic cancer risks has revealed a high risk for a given participant—it is suggested the researcher simply needs to know when to doff her "researcher" hat and to put (back) on her physician hat.[2] In the context of ancillary-care issues, however, there are several reasons why this sort of response fails. First, while the case of clinicians who recruit their patients into drug trials illustrates how it can come about that one individual genuinely relates to one research participant both as that person's physician and as the (or an) investigator in a study in which that person is participating,

---

2. A particularly sophisticated version of this idea is developed in Resnik (2009). I note that Resnik's goal is to develop an overall account of the ethics of clinical research, whereas my goal here is simply to develop an account of the special ancillary-care obligation applying to medical researchers. For the latter purpose, at least, it is important to postpone the contextualism a bit so as to be able first to articulate a clear position.

this sort of case is by no means typical. There are many other ways in which research participants may be recruited. Even sticking with drug trials in industrialized countries, it is plain that an overlap between the roles of personal physician and drug researcher is not that likely. More commonly, personal physicians refer their patients to the researchers. In contexts such as that of malaria trials funded in developing countries by national research institutes such as the U.S. National Institutes of Health or by NGOs such as the Gates Foundation, say, such an overlap is even less likely. Instead, in those cases, the researchers often are present in a community only for the duration of the study and do not otherwise play any major role in taking on patients.

A second reason the "two hats" response is inadequate is that, in many cases of medical research, the research team is made up primarily of non-physicians. In the Malaria Researchers and Schistosomiasis case, the principal investigators might be Ph.D. parasitologists rather than physicians. To be sure, one might dispute what counts as "medical research." Because the moral grounds for the partial-entrustment model, as explained in the following chapter, do not particularly hang on the demarcation of medical research from other forms of research, I follow a broad understanding of "medical research" here. Obviously, we are here concerned with medical research involving human beings. I will understand "medical research involving human beings" to be any kind of scientific research that enrolls human participants and that concerns itself with the workings of the human body. On this definition, "medical research" (as I will call it, for short) will include the case of Brain Scans, mentioned in the previous chapter, even though such a trial is likely to be conducted by cognitive scientists with training in psychology or even philosophy, rather than by physicians. I recognize that this broad use of the term "medical research" strains ordinary usage. I do not mean thereby to be particularly provocative;

rather, it is just that I know of no better term to cover the range of cases I have in mind. ("Somatic research" might do, but has the disadvantage of being an unfamiliar coinage.) The substantive point will be that the cognitive scientists conducting the experiment in Brain Scans can accrue a special ancillary-care obligation whose content and basis is of a piece with that accrued by physicians running a drug trial.[3]

Finally, the most basic problem with the "two hats" response to the ancillary-care issue is that it leaves medical researchers without any clear guidance. The unacceptability of the two polar responses to the issue does tell us that it will be morally inadequate to approach the issue either solely as an idealized physician or solely as a blinkered scientist. There is nothing in the role morality of the situation, however, that indicates in any more fine-grained way how individuals occupying the intermediate role of a medical researcher working with human subjects—or individuals occupying both the role of a scientific researcher and the role of a clinician with respect to a given participant—can make an acceptable hybrid of the two "pure" roles of physician and scientist. They certainly cannot reasonably do so simply by alternating between them as the circumstances seem to dictate. What makes ancillary-care issues so troubling in many cases is that roles of *both* types apply simultaneously. The medical researcher needs some guidance in coping with this conflict. The conflict cannot be evaded by pretending that one side of it either disappears or is somehow overridden by a higher commitment, whether to the physician's Hippocratic ideal or to the scientist's pursuit of general knowledge. What researchers need is some principled guidance about their ancillary-care

---

3. One might consider also the case of public-health researchers: see Richardson (2010) and Hyder & Merritt (2009). I do not mean to minimize the relevant differences among these different forms of research, and will return to them in the penultimate chapter. For now, however, I will continue to use the term "medical research" capaciously.

obligations, not simply a statement that it is up to them to decide how to deal with this conflict.

Let us focus, then, on the in-between role of medical researchers working with human subjects. If we look to existing understandings of the ethics of this profession and existing guidelines that apply to it, we will find, as I have mentioned, that these do not speak to the issue of ancillary care. What we will instead discover is that these materials simply serve to reproduce and reinforce the conflicts that cry out for more guidance. Hence, on the one side, the introduction of the World Medical Association's Declaration of Helsinki, as revised in 2008, states that "It is the duty of the physician to promote and safeguard the health of patients, including those who are involved in medical research."⁴ No one, however, takes this to require researchers—even physician-researchers—to do everything in their power to promote the health of their research participants. The participants in the Georgetown workshop make this point with the following example (Participants, 2008, 1–2):

> Physician–researchers who seek to follow this dictum will encounter difficulties when their participants in a medically underserved area develop health needs that outstrip the research team's resources or plans; for example, when a rural participant in a study of vitamin A deficiency is found to have cancer treatable only at the tertiary-care hospital in the capital of the neighboring country. Taking the Helsinki dictum directly to generate ancillary-care obligations would yield an unreasonably expansive requirement.

In truth, the statement from the introduction to the Declaration of Helsinki was not meant to provide direct guidance, but rather

---

4. For a slightly fuller rundown of existing guidelines that speak to areas adjacent to ancillary care, at least, see Participants (2008, 1). I am grateful to Christine Grady for help in locating relevant guidelines.

a general orientation. Given the unacceptability of the polar positions, it is too vague to address the ancillary-care issue in any helpful way.

Further, at least many medical researchers work under restrictions imposed by their funders that run in the other direction. For example, researchers funded by the U.S. National Institutes of Health (NIH) are restricted by a policy of the Inspector General of the Department of Health and Human Services, according to which no NIH research funds are to be used for medical care that is not "study-related." The NIH is not alone in this (Philpott et al., 2010). These sorts of policies, like the statement from the Declaration of Helsinki quoted in the last paragraph, are quite vague. What is "study-related"? Clearly, however, they push in the opposite direction, making it difficult for researchers funded by these entities to provide any ancillary care. Many researchers working in developing countries seem simply to find ways around this limit. In the case of NIH practice, for instance, while funds are not to be used for "care," they may be used to build and stock a clinic in the study location. That is because the NIH limitation was imposed not out of concern about the potentially spiraling costs of providing ancillary care in developing countries, but out of concern about politicians in Washington taking advantage of the proximity of NIH's world-class research hospital to get free, state-of-the-art medical care there for themselves and their family members. It is ironic that a limitation that was imposed for this reason is now interfering with the provision of ancillary care to destitute study participants in the poorest countries of the world.

That this is unfortunate has at least been recognized in the ethics guidelines of the Council for International Organizations of Medical Sciences (CIOMS, 2002). In the commentary to Guideline 21, CIOMS states that "although sponsors are, in general, not obliged to provide health care services beyond what is necessary for the conduct of research, it is morally praiseworthy to do so." Yet we have already seen that, as far as ancillary care is concerned, this statement does not go far enough. *Some* instances of providing ancillary care are not merely morally praiseworthy, but morally obligatory.[5]

If this is admitted, then there would actually be a way of reconciling the provision of ancillary care with limitations such as the Inspector General's. As I have noted, the term "study-related" is quite vague. "Study-related" expenses are routinely recognized as including expenses whose necessity derives not from science, but from the ethical requirements relevant to medical research. For instance, obtaining informed consent is often quite difficult and expensive, but research sponsors do not balk at spending funds to obtain duly informed consent. They recognize that this expense is "study-related." It is related to the study because it is part of what is morally required in order to proceed permissibly with the study. If it were similarly recognized that the provision of some ancillary care were also morally required in order to proceed permissibly with a study, then, by the same argument, spending on ancillary care would also count as "study-related."[6]

---

5. Miller, Mello, and Joffe (2008, p. 278) write that "Though perhaps praiseworthy, providing nonemergency follow-up care is not an obligation that arises from the nature of the researchers' professional relationship with subjects." They do not there give any arguments for this position, however. My full argument for the stronger position that an obligation—albeit a *pro tanto* or defeasible one—arises will be set out only in the following chapter.

6. Compare the parallel point made by Miller, Mello, and Joffe (2008), 278. It might be objected that "study-related" has a stricter meaning when applied to the provision of medical care than when applied to consent procedures. In answer to this, I note that in some cases, it is necessary to provide medical care in order to obtain meaningful informed consent. For instance, a potential participant delirious with fever must first be stabilized before his or her informed consent can meaningfully be solicited. Hence, even if we focus on the provision of medical care, existing practices of obtaining informed consent show that what is "study-related" includes what is related to the study by virtue of ethical requirements.

Having just argued from the premise that there are ancillary-care obligations, I should pause to clarify what I mean. My point here is a narrow one. It is that, *sometimes*, the provision of ancillary care is not merely morally praiseworthy, but morally obligatory. To say this is not to assert a general or blanket ancillary-care obligation, one that holds in all circumstances. As a practical matter, it may be that the most important message that needs to be gotten across is simply that researchers, research sponsors, IRBs, and RECs need to try to anticipate ancillary-care needs that may arise in research and consider how best to address them. I will return to these practical matters in the final chapter. For now, however, in working towards a philosophically adequate articulation of researchers' ancillary-care obligations, the point we seem to have reached is that *there are some*, even if it is difficult, in advance, to specify the conditions under which this is so.[7]

But if existing understandings of the profession of medical research and existing guidelines addressed to that profession do not provide any help in indicating the scope and limits of ancillary-care obligations, where are we to find relevant guidance? What answer does the partial-entrustment model offer? As a first step, its suggestion is that we must work harder to understand the still ill-understood intermediate role of the medical researcher working on human subjects. The partial-entrustment model suggests that we will understand this role better if we take a closer look at the process whereby particular researchers and research teams come to have a researcher–participant relationship with particular individuals: the process of obtaining participants' informed consent. The attention that has been lavished on informed consent has, to date, all been driven by quite different sorts of questions: questions

---

7. Here, I am attempting to respond to thoughtful objections raised by Malcolm Molyneux.

about the avoidance of exploitation, the autonomy of participants, the possibility of permissibly enrolling children or the mentally disabled, and the like. Once we look at the informed-consent process from the perspective of potential ancillary-care obligations, however, quite a different perspective opens up.

## SCOPE: PARTIAL ENTRUSTMENT OF ASPECTS OF HEALTH

According to the partial-entrustment model, the special ancillary-care obligation is limited in scope. It applies only to a proper subset of needs for ancillary care. As I have mentioned, this has proven to be the most controversial aspect of the partial-entrustment account. Yet insofar as those dissatisfied with the proposal's particular scope limitation still aim to articulate a special obligation that researchers owe to their research participants, the onus on them is to provide an alternative account of what it is about the relationship between researcher and participant that grounds a broader obligation. As to general obligations, such as the duty of beneficence or the duty of rescue, I remind the reader that the special ancillary-care obligation put forward by the partial-entrustment model is naturally seen as *supplementing* any such general obligations, which are commonly seen as being too weak to require significant diversion of resources away from otherwise permissible projects such as the conduct of sound medical research.[8]

---

8. I offer no general account of how to settle conflicts of prioritization that might arise when the duty of rescue pulls one way and the special ancillary-care obligation pulls another. Merritt (2011, 331) seems to suggest that my presentation of the partial-entrustment model in terms of a two-stage model of deliberation suggests otherwise, but the conclusion of that deliberation is only that there is (or is not) a special ancillary-care obligation. It is not a conclusion about all-things-considered obligation.

Let us turn, then, to the process that establishes a researcher–participant relationship, namely the process of obtaining potential participants' informed consent to participate in a study. In light of the concerns that have dominated research ethics to date, the informed-consent process is seen as serving two morally important functions:

1. (*non-exploitation*) to provide a check against exploitation by ensuring that important facts about the study, including any known risks, are shared between researchers and potential participants before the study begins
2. (*autonomy*) to help ensure that participants' decisions to enroll in a study are not only not manipulated, coerced, or ignorant but reflect their autonomous responses to a reasonably well-informed understanding of the nature of the study

The first of these functions views the informed-consent process as being a procedural check on a par with review by an IRB or REC. Such procedural checks are seen as being important to help ensure that nothing remotely similar to the kind of abuse that occurred in the Tuskegee Syphilis Study ever occurs again. The second of these functions is somewhat more ambitious or aspirational, and enshrines in medical research ethics a principle parallel to that of patient autonomy in clinical medicine. That is, it places special value on the individual participant making up his or her own mind about whether to participate, without being unduly influenced even by the sincere and factually sound arguments of the researchers. There is now much debate about how much stress to lay on this second role of informed consent (e.g., Sreenivasan, 2003; Kukla, 2005; Miller & Wertheimer, 2007). Interesting as it is, this debate does not concern us, for the function of informed consent central to the partial-entrustment model is a third, more basic one, distinct from both the exploitation-avoiding function and the autonomy-promoting function.

Even apart from any special need to avoid exploitation or to promote participant autonomy, it would still be necessary for medical researchers to obtain potential participants' consent. The reason for this, generically, is that participants in medical research are asked to waive some of their rights to privacy. Albeit with some local variations, it is universally recognized that rights of privacy attach to individuals' bodies, bodily functions, and medical histories (CIOMS, 2002, Guideline 5.14).[9] Because medical researchers need to collect information about their participants' bodies, bodily functions, and medical histories, they need to obtain prospective participants' permission to do so. Proceeding to touch the participants, gather blood samples from them, and pore over their medical histories without having obtained permission to do so, first, would in general be impermissible.[10] Hence, the third function of obtaining informed consent, largely neglected in the bioethics literature, is the following:

3. (*permission-obtaining*) to obtain prospective participants' permission to examine their bodies, study their bodily functions, and collect their medical histories, in the ways required by the study

---

9. For a more detailed discussion of these privacy rights, see Chapter 3.
10. One exception allowed for by the "in general" hedge concerns emergency-medicine research (cf. Emanuel, Wendler, & Grady, 2000). Another, arguably, is that doing research on stored biological samples does not require first obtaining specific permission from the individuals from whom the samples were obtained, provided that they were obtained with permission. Ellen Wright Clayton (2005) stresses that, under current practice in the United States, researchers using banked samples often have no relation to the individuals from whom the samples were obtained. If these individuals had not given permission for later researchers to use the samples, however, the later research may be morally faulted, it seems to me, on privacy grounds. I return to the issue of biobank research in the penultimate chapter, as it raises fascinating issues about the bounds of the researcher–participant relationship.

Whereas the exploitation-avoiding function of informed consent casts it as instrumental to avoiding an evil and the autonomy-promoting function casts it as serving an independent moral requirement or aspiration, the permission-obtaining function of informed consent is essential to getting the researcher–participant relationship up and running (Table 2). If we are to understand the researcher–participant relationship as a morally acceptable one to which certain special obligations might attach, we need to understand it as being built on the participants' freely given permissions—on their having consented, in the informed-consent process, to relaxing their privacy rights in the ways necessary for the trial to go forward in permissible fashion.

Understanding the researcher–participant relationship in this way, the partial-entrustment model sees the special ancillary-care obligation as resulting from this process whereby the researchers obtain the permissions they need to go forward. The *scope* of the special ancillary-care obligation, according to the partial-entrustment model, is determined by the set of permissions that the researchers had to have obtained in order to proceed permissibly with their study. The actual set of permissions gathered in

Table 2. FUNCTIONS OF OBTAINING INFORMED
CONSENT FROM RESEARCH PARTICIPANTS

| FUNCTION | HOW ACHIEVED? |
| --- | --- |
| 1. Avoiding exploitation | Informed-consent process as a procedural check |
| 2. Promoting autonomy | By involving participants in choice |
| 3. Obtaining permission | By obtaining waivers of privacy rights |

a given study's informed-consent process may, in fact, be too narrow—because the documents fail to mention procedures for which permission should be obtained—or, more commonly, too broad—because, say, the lawyers have gotten involved and have written language whereby those who agree to participate give very broad, blanket permissions, beyond what is necessary to carry out the study in question. For these reasons, the set of permissions actually obtained is not what matters for determining the scope of the special ancillary-care obligation. Instead, what matters is the set of permissions that, given the study design, had to have been gathered for the researchers to avoid violating the participants' privacy rights.

The central claim of the partial-entrustment model is that, simply by providing researchers with these special permissions, participants effectively entrust the researchers with special responsibilities to look after needs they discover by acting on those permissions. By the same token, by accepting the participants' needed permissions, the researchers become effectively entrusted with such special responsibilities.[11] This entrustment comes about not because either of the parties thinks that such entrustment is going on—quite probably, neither does—but (for reasons I will explain

11. In this claim, the version of a partial-entrustment model advanced here is in basic agreement with the one developed, drawing on my work with Belsky, by Miller, Mello, and Joffe (2008). They, too, stress the moral relevance of the fact the medical research trucks in private information—information to which privacy rights normally apply—and take this to be central to determining what is entrusted to researchers by research participants. I here ignore a stray remark they make at p. 278 about the bodies also being entrusted to the researchers ("the researcher-subject relationship involves investigator access to and entrustment with subjects' private information and their bodies, pursuant to subjects' consent to participate in the research study"). I take it that what they mean is that the researchers have been given "privileged access" to the participants' bodies because the participants have given them permission, in the informed-consent process, to have such access, thereby waiving their rights to privacy. Just such an informational and privacy-rights–based account was put forward in my own contribution to that same special issue of the *Journal of Law, Medicine, and Ethics* (Richardson, 2008a).

in the following chapter) as a result of the participants' waiving their privacy rights. For example, since the researchers in Malaria Researchers and Schistosomiasis needed to have obtained permission to look at their participants' fluid samples under a microscope, they are thereby entrusted with special responsibilities in relation to other things they discover in so doing, such as schistosomes in the participants' blood or urine. Since the researchers in Brain Scans needed to have obtained permission to look at scans of their participants' brains, they are thereby entrusted with special responsibilities in relation to things they see in so doing. Again, I postpone until the following chapter a proper philosophical *defense* of this central claim of the partial-entrustment model.[12] Here, my task is to expound the model.

Anticipating the account to be offered in the following chapter, I suggest that the reader understand the permission-obtaining function of the informed-consent process as serving to shift certain responsibilities from the participants to the researchers. As a default matter, most adults have primary responsibility for looking after their own health. What the partial-entrustment model asserts is this: By giving special permission to the researchers to probe their bodies, examine their bodily functions, and interrogate their medical histories, research participants delegate some responsibility for certain aspects of their health to the researchers. Which aspects of their health? The ones covered by the permissions needed for the study to proceed permissibly.

Let me offer four comments about this proposal about the scope of entrustment underlying the special ancillary-care obligation. First, in the preceding paragraphs, I have been speaking

---

12. The following chapter's appeal to the idea of moral entanglement supersedes our earlier appeal to the relevance of compassion, engagement, and gratitude (Richardson & Belsky, 2004, 28), which is subject to searching criticism in Wertheimer (2011, 277–279).

of "responsibilities," not "obligations." According to the partial-entrustment model, being within the scope of the obligation is just the first of two necessary conditions for an ancillary-care obligation to arise. The strength of a purported claim to ancillary care must also be assessed before any obligation can be assigned.

Second, the preceding paragraphs have already said what I *mean* by "entrustment." Generically, to entrust someone with something is to delegate to him or her certain special responsibilities regarding it. The central claim of the partial-entrustment model is that research participants do this *by* giving the researchers special permissions that relax privacy rights. Again, at the risk of being boringly repetitive, I note that it will be the task of the next chapter to defend this central claim. As long as it is understood that this is my claim, however, it should be clear that when I write about "entrustment" I am *not* making any claim either about (a) what the participants are *explicitly doing* when they sign up for studies or (b) what the participants or the researchers *believe or expect*. The claim is not that the participants, in effect, *say* to the researchers, "I hereby entrust to you certain aspects of my health." That claim would be absurd, for research participants do not do this. Further, the claim is not that the beliefs or expectations of the participants—or of the researchers—settle anything morally. While many research participants do expect researchers to provide them medical care, this is widely regarded as problematic: as evincing or exacerbating the so-called "therapeutic misconception" (Appelbaum et al., 1987). One set of critics has objected on this ground to the position that Belsky and I took on the Brain Scans case, which was that researchers likely have an affirmative obligation to read the scans diagnostically or to obtain diagnostic-quality scans (Miller, Mello, & Joffe, 2008, 278). In investigating researchers' ancillary-care obligations, I am in a limited way investigating a special case in which participants' expectations that the researchers should provide them some care would, in fact, sometimes be justified. As I see it, however, for these expectations to be justified, there must be a justification for the claim that the researchers have an ancillary-care obligation towards them—a justification that stands independently of those expectations. The partial-entrustment model does not build the special ancillary-care obligation on any such expectations but rather on a type of implicit entrustment of which the parties may well be unaware.

Third, the scope of entrustment is defined objectively, on the basis of the nature of the study. This is a corollary of the last point, which was that the scope of entrustment is not defined on a subjective basis, by reference to the states of mind of the participants or the researchers. This point is very important practically, for it means that IRBs and RECs may look to a study's protocol, which they must approve prior to research on human subjects being done, as a sufficient and objective basis for indicating the scope of the potential ancillary-care claims arising from that study. The protocol will indicate in what ways the researchers will need to probe the participants' bodies, track their bodily functions, and ascertain their medical histories. These are the activities for which the researchers need the participants' special permission, and these permissions are what set the scope of the special ancillary-care obligation. Accordingly, on the partial-entrustment account, the scope of this special obligation rests on an objective basis that is open to objective scrutiny, not only in principle, but also in practice.

Finally, we must beware of taking too concretely talk of the participants' entrusting certain "aspects" of their health to the researchers. What set the scope of the entrustment are the permissions, and the permissions are permissions to *do* certain things: to examine a participant's body and its functions in certain ways or to collect information about a participant's medical history.[13]

---

13. The remainder of this paragraph is taken from Richardson (2008a).

A different sort of partial-entrustment model, which I reject, might generate a different answer—for example, a partial-entrustment model according to which "aspects" of a person's health, thought of as being almost a kind of "thing," are entrusted to the researchers' care. For instance, one might think that participants in an emphysema study entrust the health of their *lungs* to the researchers' care (or is it their respiratory system more generally?). For someone proceeding down this route, the tendency would be to let the boundaries of the entrustment be set either by the boundaries of our major organs or else by the conventional boundaries of medical specialties. On the latter basis, a participant in an ear-infection study might be thought to entrust to the researchers the care of his ear, nose, and throat. This crudely reified and body-based idea of the scope of entrustment is not the one that our partial-entrustment model endorses.[14] Instead, on the account I defend, the scope of entrustment is keyed to the *procedures*—understood broadly so as to include taking medical histories, doing physical exams, running scans, administering drugs, and otherwise intervening—that the research protocol prescribes.

Therefore, the scope limitation on the special ancillary-care obligation that the partial-entrustment model defends both reflects the way that researcher–participant relationships are formed in the first place and gives us a practically useful way to delimit appeals to this special obligation. Of course, stepping back from the partial-entrustment model to the broader issue it is meant to address, we had already seen that any appropriate account of ancillary-care duties will delimit such claims in some

---

14. The analogy to the old common-law idea of bailment in Richardson & Belsky (2004) has the disadvantage that it may suggest this reified interpretation of the scope of entrustment, since bailment is the limited entrustment of some valuable *thing*, such as an automobile. Our intention, however, was simply to use this analogy to introduce the idea of a limited and partial entrustment. The appeal to this analogy is now superseded by the considerations set out in the following chapter.

way. The partial-entrustment model delimits them by the tests of scope and strength. Falling outside the scope of the special ancillary-care obligation, as interpreted by the partial-entrustment model, will be care for diseases or conditions whose presence is sufficiently obvious or open to view that no special permission is required to discover them. One example of a condition outside the scope of the partial-entrustment obligation is a limb deformity resulting from a badly set broken bone—a condition unfortunately all too common in developing countries, where a subset of such problems is blandly referred to under the heading of "road accident sequelae." Many such deformities are obvious to the naked eye. Some of them—especially those that cause limps and otherwise interfere with mobility—would in developed countries be treated by rebreaking and resetting the bones. Some research teams would have the capacity to do such an operation. Yet because these problems are visible to the naked eye, and thus would be detected by someone with a trained eye without having to act on any special permissions, addressing such problems falls outside the scope of the partial-entrustment obligation (see Richardson & Belsky, 2004, 32). An example of a disease whose presence would fall outside the scope of the special ancillary-care obligation for the same reason is a dental disease, such as advanced gingivitis (see Belsky & Richardson, 2004, 1495). In such cases, the individual has only to open his or her mouth for the presence of the disease to be plain. To dramatize the issue, one can imagine that this revelation occurs even before any of the informed-consent process has begun—so, before the researcher–participant relationship has been established. According to the partial-entrustment view, a researcher's obligations in such a case are essentially the same as a researcher's obligations regarding the advanced gingivitis he or she sees in the lady selling spices in the local market.

This is not to say that these obligations are nil. As I stressed in the opening chapter, the principal target of my analysis is the special ancillary-care obligation, which supplements general obligations that all of us have. If a tropical disease specialist strolling through a local market sees a baby that seems plainly feverish with what is surely malaria, she arguably has a rescue-based duty to give the baby's mother some of the drugs she happens to be carrying and to instruct her on their use. Or, perhaps better, she could tell the mother to come immediately to the research clinic, if there is one. Researchers working in developing countries, in particular, are surrounded by all sorts of moral claims upon their attention and efforts. We need to sort out the various different ones. It makes sense to begin, as one team of researchers conducting cluster-randomized public health trials in Bangladesh, India, Malawi, and Nepal recently put it, with "a duty of care for people...when data collection teams identify risks to health" (Osrin et al., 2009, 777). The partial-entrustment model's scope restriction, which builds on what researchers find out when carrying out study procedures, whatever they are, is essential to its attempt to delineate a special ancillary-care obligation.

## THE VARIABLE STRENGTH OF ANCILLARY-CARE CLAIMS

In the terminology I have been using, the fact that a potential or purported claim for ancillary care falls within the scope of the special ancillary-care obligation means that the researchers may very well have an obligation to provide or arrange such care. Whether the researchers actually do have an obligation to provide such care, however, or to arrange for its provision (e.g., by providing "assisted referrals" [Barsdorf et al., 2010, 85])—intuitively seems to depend on a range of other contextual factors. These are factors that emerge from discussions with researchers and patient advocates as being highly relevant to such claims, as well as having an intelligible connection to a recognized moral consideration. Ideally, it might be desirable to have a more unified view of the special ancillary-care obligation, on which such contextual factors were more integrated into the core account of the obligation's scope. Such a fully integrated view, however, seems at present conceptually out of reach, and may, in any case, prove too controversial to be of practical use. At least for now, then, I content myself with retaining the two-part nature of the partial-entrustment view as originally presented, with its tiered tests of scope and strength.

Assuming that the scope requirement is met, the contextual factors affecting the strength of a specific ancillary-care obligation— or, otherwise put, of a participant's specific claim for ancillary care—most prominently include the following:

(a) (*vulnerability*) How much difference would getting the care in question make to the health or welfare of the participant?

(b) (*dependence*) How dependent is the participant on the research team for getting that care?

(c) (*engagement*) How expectably intense and long-lived is the relationship between researcher and participant, as defined by the study?

(d) (*gratitude*) Do the researchers owe the participant any debt of gratitude for his or her willingness to have undergone procedures that are risky, painful, or inconvenient?

(e) (*cost*) Countervailingly, what is the cost to the research enterprise (in terms of budget, personnel time, and the ability to gather clear and statistically significant data) of providing any ancillary care?

Gratitude was mentioned in the first chapter; the other elements of the test of strength call for some further elaboration.

The most obvious and most obviously relevant aspect of these dimensions of strength is the contest between what I am here calling "vulnerability" on one side and "cost" on the other. As the examples already given make plain, getting needed ancillary care can often make a huge difference—indeed, a life-or-death difference—to a research participant. Yet, as was also plain from the very first discussions of ancillary-care issues in the context of planned HIV-vaccine trials, the provision of needed ancillary care can be very costly, and indeed can represent a level of cost that would swamp the relevant research budget.

One might question why cost counts as a morally relevant feature. To take an example familiar in moral philosophy, we would normally consider it wrong, or a sign of moral vice, for someone to pause before rescuing a drowning child on account of the costliness of the silk suit he will ruin in so doing.[15] More generally, when a person is in urgent peril, and one could save the person, stopping to worry about the costs of saving the person may seem inappropriate. Why, then, take cost to be a factor affecting the strength of the special ancillary-care obligation in specific circumstances? There are two answers to this question. First, although, as I have said, I am not in a position to provide a fully integrated account of ancillary-care obligations, it would not be implausible to suppose that such a fully integrated account would *mention* considerations of cost. That this is a plausible possibility can be seen by analogy to the principle of rescue. In a way that is hardly unusual, T. M. Scanlon (1998, 224) states a "rescue principle" incorporating considerations of cost,

---

15. "Normally," only. If, as in Liam Murphy's version of such a story, the agent's reason for pausing in this way is that he is considering how many more lives he would save by doing some fundraising for OXFAM while wearing this, his only suit, then matters are different (Murphy, 2000, 129).

as follows: "if you are presented with a situation in which you can prevent something very bad from happening, or alleviate someone's dire plight, by making only a slight (or even moderate) sacrifice, then it would be wrong not to do so." Here, the idea of "sacrifice" serves to capture the idea of the costs to the agent of providing needed aid. It would make sense for a fully integrated ancillary-care principle to do so as well. Since we are not in a position to state a fully integrated ancillary-care principle, it makes sense instead to flag cost as a factor affecting the strength of a claim that falls within the scope of the obligation.

The second reason that it makes moral sense to include consideration of cost is that, generally speaking, medical research is a socially valuable enterprise. With this in mind, the cost factor as stated above focuses on the costs *to science* of providing ancillary care. For such costs, the immediate costs to a given study team must serve as the only practicable proxy. Independent moral grounds rule out conducting medical research on human beings that is *not* socially valuable. As Emanuel, Wendler, and Grady (2000, 2703) state,

> To be ethical, clinical research must be valuable, meaning that it evaluates a diagnostic or therapeutic intervention that could lead to improvements in health or well-being; is a preliminary etiological, pathophysiological, or epidemiological study to develop such an intervention; or tests a hypothesis that can generate important knowledge about structure or function of human biological systems, even if that knowledge does not have immediate practical ramifications.

In the present context, in developing an account of ancillary-care obligations, I hope I will be forgiven for idealizing and simplifying to the extent of assuming that this requirement of social value is met by the studies in question. If a trial does not meet this requirement, then the primary point is that it should not be conducted, not that those conducting it should provide more ancillary care. A similar point applies to research that unduly exploits those in developing countries.[16] Assuming, then, that the research in question is both socially valuable in this sense and is otherwise morally permissible, one must worry about burdening this socially valuable enterprise with undue costs.

In summarizing the strength-affecting factors, I distinguished several aspects of cost. Although the monetary and personnel costs are relatively obvious, even they deserve some comment. It is reasonable to worry about the magnitude of the monetary cost of providing a given sort of ancillary care. In considering this issue, however, we must not take for granted that research budgets are fixed. Perhaps it is morally incumbent on those funding medical research—including, ultimately, such bodies as the U.S. Congress, which appropriates the funds for the NIH—to take ancillary-care obligations into account in making research funds available. Perhaps it is morally incumbent on the more immediate sponsors of research to build some funds for ancillary care into their research grants. Even so, as the last chapter's example of HIV-vaccine trials illustrated, there are limits to what even the best-intentioned can accomplish along these lines. About costs in terms of personnel time, we should simply take note of why this element is worth separating out, in that in many parts of the world, and especially in developing countries, trained personnel capable of undertaking medical research are extremely scarce. There is also an element of cost that concerns the generation of data. As a theoretical matter, it seems possible in many contexts that provision of ancillary care

---

16. I will return to the important questions raised by the issue of exploitation in Chapter 4.

could either make the data more difficult to interpret or else require the investigators to drop the participant in question from the study—a move that might have unfortunate consequences in, say, a study of a disease or condition rare enough that only a few individuals qualified for the study in the first place. Such effects might make it more difficult for the researchers to generate statistically significant results. It has proven difficult to find clear examples of these effects, however, in part because in many types of investigations, such as drug trials, researchers are already used to tracking and taking account of "adverse events" of highly varied kinds. They tend to be proud of their ability to generate significant data despite these difficulties. Nonetheless, we should remain alert to this possible type of cost.

The important issue of the researchers' *ability* to provide or arrange for the needed ancillary care is largely subsumed under the dimension of cost. Where ancillary-care needs can be anticipated, additional specialists could be hired to broaden a research team's ability to meet those needs more easily. Where an ancillary-care need does arise that the team cannot handle, they nonetheless often *could* med-evac the person to a hospital that could provide the needed care. It is just that doing so would be very expensive. If they truly cannot do anything to help the person, then, by the general ethical principle that "ought" implies "can," they have no obligation to do so. Despite this considerable overlap with the dimension of cost, the dimension of *ability*—including the important element of competence or expertise—is worthy of attention and something that our earlier presentations of the partial-entrustment model did not adequately stress.[17]

The concept picked out by the "vulnerability" factor should not pose any problem, although the terminology might mislead some.

17. Resnik (2009), p. 7 of online version, drew this issue to my attention.

The point is not to pick out some individuals as vulnerable, absolutely speaking. Rather, the idea is to identify respects in which participants' health and/or welfare is *vulnerable to* how others act, and specifically to whether or not they receive aid in the form of ancillary care.[18] It might be thought criticizably imprecise to fail to choose between effects on welfare and effects on health or to indicate how to measure trade-offs between health and non-health aspects of welfare. This criticism expects more precision here than may reasonably be demanded. We can recognize that the effects of untreated schistosomiasis and neglected brain tumors can be very serious, without needing to compare their relative seriousness. Since we are discussing an obligation specially incumbent on individual medical researchers (or medical research teams), there is no great call for a centralized system for allocating resources to ancillary care based on their comparative seriousness.

If vulnerability, in this sense, is an indication of the degree of difference it would make to an individual whether or not he or she receives a given sort of ancillary care, "dependence" is an indication of the degree to which the individual's hopes for getting ancillary care hang on whether or not the research team provides it (or arranges for its provision). One reason that I have been, and will continue to be, focusing especially on cases from developing countries is that it is there that research participants are most likely to be highly dependent on the research teams for any access to medical care. As the United States illustrates, however, access to medical care even in some of the wealthier industrialized countries can be quite uneven. One way that I am *not* here proposing to idealize is by presuming full justice around the world in access to medical care!

18. On this relational sort of vulnerability, see, e.g., Goodin (1985, 33 and 163n.). Whereas Goodin has in mind ways in which one person is "vulnerable to" another specific person, I have left the other person unspecified in order to keep this kind of vulnerability distinct from the factor of dependence, to be discussed next.

Such an idealization would completely change the contours of the ancillary-care issue as we must face it.[19]

The final element of the strength of ancillary-care claims is the degree of "engagement." This is a rough gauge of the depth of the human relationship that will be forged between members of the research team and individual participants during the course of a study. In a long-term observational study of inpatients who are suffering a rare and ill-understood disease, the degree of engagement will be extremely high. In a study that involves a one-time interaction with participants in order to collect a biological sample—say, by swabbing the inside of their cheeks—the degree of engagement will be extremely low. Intuitively, the level of human interaction between researchers and participants seems to make a difference to how much the researchers owe the participants. The longer and deeper their interaction, the harder it will be for the researchers to deny needed ancillary care without seeming to imply that they are treating the participants as mere means to gathering data. This, at least, is a rough psychological fact, and it is one to which many give moral importance. In thinking about the factor of engagement, however, we must be careful to steer clear of morally arbitrary factors that arise in the same ballpark. It is presumably not relevant to the strength of a given claim for ancillary care whether the participant and the researcher *like* each other or otherwise get along. Similarly, it will not be relevant whether they have spent hours in the hospital cafeteria chatting about life. What matters, as indicated above, is the intensity and the duration of their interaction, *as this may be predicted on the basis of the study protocol*. In other words, at least as a first approximation, to assess the morally relevant aspect

19. A philosopher such as the late G. A. Cohen might argue that this shows that the ancillary-care principles articulated here are not fundamental ethical principles, but rather are "fact-dependent" principles: see Cohen (2008). To the contrary, I would argue that any ethical principle worthy of the name is fact-dependent, in Cohen's sense.

of the personal engagement between participant and researcher, we should look to the ways in which the design of the study requires that they interact. By the "intensity" of their interaction, I have in mind such features as whether their interaction involves a series of outpatient visits (less intense) or an equivalent amount of time that the participant spends as an inpatient (more intense). Being in intensive care involves more intense interactions than does being on an ordinary ward for observation. And so on.

## COMBINING THE TESTS OF SCOPE AND STRENGTH

According to the partial-entrustment model, researchers have a special ancillary-care obligation to provide (or arrange for the provision of) ancillary care of a given kind only if the participant's claim to it meets both the test of scope and the test of strength. The test of scope is relatively precise: one must determine whether or not the researchers' knowledge of the need in question arose (or would have arisen[20]) from carrying out study procedures. The test of strength is not precise, nor should one attempt to make it so; still—as I shall argue more at length in Chapter 6—one may approach the strength issues systematically. IRBs and RECs, for instance, would be able to make reasoned comparisons of the relative strength of two different claims for ancillary care. Still, the test of strength will remain a matter of judgment. However this may be, the partial-entrustment model holds that a participant has a special ancillary-care claim if

---

20. Suppose that the malaria researcher in Malaria Researchers and Schistosomiasis had already heard from his brother-in-law that a given participant was suffering from schistosomiasis. Still, care for schistosomiasis falls within the scope of the special ancillary-care obligation, as I propose to interpret it, as carrying out the study procedures would almost surely have revealed this fact to the researcher.

and only if the claim given is both within the scope and sufficiently strong to be honored.

This simple position can be put in graphic terms in (see Figure 1).

In later chapters, I will go into the tests of scope and strength in detail. The following chapter will address the crucial limitation of scope, while Chapter 6 will illustrate in detail how the strength test may be used in practice. To illustrate the sort of case in which an ancillary-care obligation would arise, however, we may return to the Malaria Researchers and Schistosomiasis case. As I have already noted, the participants' claim to ancillary care for schistosomiasis in that case is within the scope of the partial-entrustment obligation, since researchers become aware of the schistosomiasis by carrying out a study procedure. The claim for at least some schistosomiasis care is also sufficiently strong, in that the population is one with little other access to medical care and the drugs to treat

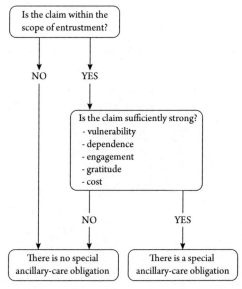

Figure 1. The Partial-Entrustment Model's Two Tests (Reproduced with permission of BMJ Publishing Group, Ltd.)

the symptoms of schistosomiasis are quite inexpensive and simple to administer.

## CONTROVERSY SURROUNDING THE SCOPE REQUIREMENT

While the various dimensions of the strength test are quite commonsensical and the strength test itself is too vague to have drawn much objection, the scope limitation built into the partial-entrustment model has been found objectionable. In a pair of articles, Neal Dickert and colleagues have argued that the scope limitation is too narrow. Since their arguments and examples pose an important challenge to the partial-entrustment view, it is worth looking at them in some detail. I start with a case involving some misunderstanding of the partial-entrustment view and then turn to a case that takes it up squarely.

The first example that Dickert and colleagues raised in questioning the scope limitation was drawn from an observational study of children with advanced malaria, the Mother-Offspring Malaria Study (MOMS) in Tanzania. As they describe the study (Dickert et al., 2007, 874), it was:

> a 5-year observational study focused on the pathogenesis and clinical outcomes of severe malarial disease in children. Participants were mother-infant pairs at the Muheza Designated District Hospital (MDDH) in Tanzania and were enrolled around the time of delivery. The protocol included obtaining peripheral, placental, and umbilical cord blood at delivery, capillary blood at 2-week intervals for the first year of life then every month until age 4 years, and venous blood every 6 months.

As the authors note, although it was being conducted in a place and time where the annual government expenditure on health was only $12/person, this study made two kinds of provision for caring for the participants. First, regular review by a co-investigator was directed towards ensuring that the participants were receiving, at study expense, appropriate inpatient and outpatient care for malaria. Second, because the study was enrolling a population in which HIV was highly prevalent, the study made provision for "hospice referral for HIV-related treatment, including co-trimoxazole prophylaxis" (874). It was, however, judged to be unfeasible to offer either treatment for the opportunistic infections to which the AIDS sufferers were prone or to provide antiretrovirals.

Commenting on this example, Dickert and colleagues suggest that in this case the HIV care fell outside the scope of the special ancillary-care obligation set out by the partial-entrustment model. Taking this to be the case, they find fault with the scope restriction on this account.

The reason that Dickert and colleagues mistakenly see the HIV care as falling outside the scope of the special ancillary-care obligation defended by the partial-entrustment model is that they interpret this scope too narrowly. Their explanation is as follows (875):

> A duty to provide care for HIV-related illness, however, seems to fall outside the scope of entrustment. Knowledge about HIV status is one of many elements of the medical history that were relevant to investigators, but data on HIV were not generated by participation, were not central to the research question, and were available to anyone interacting clinically with participants.

Yet as these investigators realized, these participants sorely needed prophylaxis for opportunistic infections, a treatment that could be provided quite inexpensively. Dickert and colleagues comment that "We see no reason why these factors ought not to have a role in establishing the scope as well" (875).

Now, I agree that the case is a morally compelling one and that, given this, it would be desirable to develop a theory that would account for such HIV care being within the scope of entrustment. I would stress, though, that a theory is needed: Since one is talking about a novel kind of special obligation, one cannot simply *make up* a desired scope of obligation, *ad lib*, but must see if there is a principled basis for taking the scope to have one shape or another. Fortunately, however, this case provides no reason to go in search of an alternative theory, for Dickert and colleagues are mistaken in supposing that in this case the HIV care falls outside of the scope of the special ancillary-care obligation put forward by the partial-entrustment model. As I have stressed, taking someone's medical history is something that requires his or her permission. So, too—although the matter is more ambiguous and debatable— does "interacting clinically" with someone. Suppose, realistically, that it is not simply visible, absent specifically clinical interaction, that these individuals had HIV. If so, then the knowledge that they had HIV derived from interacting with them in ways that required their permission and in ways required for the study to go forward. Accordingly, their HIV and its progression did indeed fall within the scope of what was entrusted to the researchers by these participants' enrolling in the study.

Now, Dickert and colleagues quite readily admit that if the study had stratified the participants according to their HIV status, this would have made a clear case for saying that their HIV was within the scope of the special ancillary-care duty Belsky and I set out. I think the spirit of this point is correct, but suggest that the difference that this makes is one of *degree*: stratification would have made it the case that these participants' HIV was *centrally* within the scope of entrustment, whereas when knowledge of the HIV arises, as far as the study goes, only from the initial hearing of the participants' medical histories, it is only *minimally* within the scope. In Chapter 6, I will elaborate these distinctions in the degree to which the scope requirement is met and why and how they matter in practice. For the present, the point is simply that, since one cannot take someone's medical history without his or her permission, information gleaned from a medical history needed—as those in MOMS were—to carry out the research does come within the scope of what participants entrust to researchers by agreeing to participate in the study.

In another article, Dickert and Wendler (2009a) put forward a pair of cases that presents a clearer substantive challenge to the scope limitation.[21] Instancing an observational study of pulmonary hypertension done in Bamako, Mali, they mention two cases: one that actually arose that was outside the scope and another one that, had it arisen, would have been. About both of these cases, they question the appropriateness of the moral verdict offered by the partial-entrustment model. The real case is that of an infant who had been brought along by its mother, who was participating in the study. The infant was plainly suffering from a severe but treatable *Chlamydia trachomatis* eye infection, a common cause of blindness that typically causes the eyelashes painfully to grow

21. Merritt (2011, 330) echoes Dickert & Wendler's case-based objection but seems to me to put the cart before the horse in rhetorically asking, "Why should participants…accept the appeal to partial entrustment as an arbiter permitting researchers to do nothing about the needs that fall outside its scope?" (331). Of course, the scope limitation needs to be justified: that is what the following chapter aims to do. But the crucial question is, rather, on what rests the participants' claims to ancillary care? The principal answer I offer is: on the claims arising from partial entrustment. It is important and helpful to ask, as Merritt's article does more generally, what makes a position reasonable from the standpoints of the researchers and the participants; but what makes the partial-entrustment view reasonable, I suggest, is the set of arguments on which it rests. Also, as I have noted, the duty of rescue provides an additional, complementary basis for such claims.

inwards. As Dickert and Wendler rightly point out, since the nature of this infection was obvious to the trained eye, it falls outside the scope of what is entrusted to the researchers—and would do even if the infant in question were a participant in the study. The other case of this kind that they instance—a hypothetical one—is that of a child with a leg wound that has progressed to osteomyelitis, a bone infection that, if left untreated, can easily lead to the loss of the limb, if not worse. They suppose, realistically, that treatment of this bone infection would require minor surgery ("débridement") and six weeks of hospitalization. Again, because this infection would be obvious to the trained eye, it falls outside the scope of what a participant in this hypertension study entrusts to the researchers.

Neither of these cases, however, provides any clear reason to abandon the scope restriction as unsound. The eye infection is both severely threatening and easily treatable. As such, it is adequately supported by the general duty of rescue and does not need any special ancillary-care obligation in its support. The leg infection is another matter, however, since it requires some surgery and an extended inpatient stay—rather more sacrifice on the team's part than the duty of rescue may demand. As to whether the hypertension researchers have any obligation to provide this surgery, Dickert and Wendler are themselves noncommittal. Instead, while suggesting that the scope restriction be abandoned, they insist that the various factors that the partial-entrustment model gathers under the heading of the "strength" of an ancillary-care claim should be considered contextually, in the light of case-by-case variations. Accordingly, they do not simply suggest that the partial-entrustment model gets the wrong answer on this case. Rather, what they argue is that the scope restriction generates a spurious distinction between cases like the osteomyelitis case and other cases in which the strength factors are roughly the same. As a roughly comparable case, they instance a real case that arose within the malaria-pulmonary hypertension study in Mali, in which the echocardiogram required by the study revealed a "massive pericardial effusion"—a potentially dangerous and abnormal accumulation of fluid around the heart—in one of the participants. Because that was discovered by carrying out a study procedure, they are correct in noting, it was clearly within the scope of the special ancillary-care obligation the partial-entrustment model puts forward. Further, they note, these researchers felt that they ought to treat this condition, and did so. But, stressing the similar degree of involvement these researchers would have had with another participant who had presented with osteomyelitis, and noting the way in which, in presenting the partial-entrustment model, Belsky and I had emphasized the importance of engaging with each participant as a "whole person" and not simply as a source of specialized biomedical data, Dickert and Wendler urge that the difference in moral treatment implied by the scope limitation is morally arbitrary.

As I have already indicated, however, the scope limitation is not arbitrary, but is grounded in a central fact about what constitutes a relationship between researcher and participant in the first place. Dickert and Wendler's thought seems to be that ancillary-care responsibilities can somehow be grounded in the relationship between researcher and participant, thought of in a looser way. As they put it (2009a, 427):

> Ancillary care responsibilities are rooted in participant-investigator relationships and are highly contextual. Because these relationships exist with whole persons and vary greatly, and because the study question does not play a privileged role in determining the relationship, the range of conditions for which potential responsibility exists is broad and cannot be limited systematically.

In response to this alternative suggestion, my response is that we would need to be told *how* this relationship between "whole persons" gives rise to this broader set of obligations. As I noted in the previous chapter, in attempting to characterize medical researchers' ancillary-care obligations towards participants in their studies, we are looking above all to understand a special obligation—one that, presumably, does not hold between medical researchers and the people they interact with at the local market.[22] Simply invoking the fact of a "relationship" between two individuals does not suffice for this purpose. Hence, Dickert and Wendler's alternative suggestion does not yet amount to a competing theory of medical researchers' ancillary-care obligations. In the coming years, I hope that they will develop one, since this neglected issue can only benefit from vigorous debate.

In the meantime, the kind of challenge that Dickert and Wendler mount against the scope restriction does show that more needs to be said about the moral basis of the scope restriction. Yes, the scope restriction put forward by the partial-entrustment model does build on a centrally defining feature of the researcher–participant relationship, namely that this relationship gets going only once prospective participants agree to waive some of their privacy rights so that the researchers can go ahead with the study. One of the reasons that the scope limitation may have seemed arbitrary to Dickert and Wendler, among others, however, is that it is not immediately apparent why this fact—that the researcher–participant relationship is initiated by a waiver of the latter's privacy rights—should count as giving rise to special ancillary-care obligations. It is the task of the following chapter to explain why this is so.

---

22. In a brief letter to the editor of *JAMA* I replied to Dickert and Wendler to this effect (Richardson, 2009). In their reasonable and measured response, Dickert and Wendler (2009b) agreed that the onus is on them to develop an alternative theory of the basis of ancillary-care obligations. Their doing so would greatly advance discussion of this issue.

# Chapter 3

# The Moral Basis of the Partial-Entrustment Model

I have argued that a sound position on medical researchers' special ancillary-care obligations will fall in between the polar extremes: They are not nil, and they are not as unlimited as are physicians' duties to their patients.[1] Further, I have suggested that since the obligation in question is one that holds specially between researchers and their participants, one should look for a basis of this obligation in the relationship itself. In looking to the needed permissions collected in the informed-consent process, the partial-entrustment model does just that. Still, in light of objections that have arisen against the scope limitation built into the partial-entrustment model, a deeper defense of the model would be desirable. Even someone willing to believe that researchers become effectively entrusted with responsibilities regarding the relevant aspects of the participants' health might desire a fuller explanation of *why* this is so. Providing such an explanation is the task of the present chapter.

---

1. This chapter is adapted from Richardson (2012). An earlier draft of this article appeared in *Journal of Moral Philosophy*, which is published by Koninklijke Brill NV.

Before I attempt to lay out and defend this explanation, let me first give a brief preview of it. The explanation starts with three moral assumptions:

1. *Privacy Rights.* All individuals have privacy rights pertaining to their bodies, their bodily functions, and their medical histories. These rights limit others' access thereto.
2. *Duty to Warn.* When they can do so without significant cost, all individuals have a duty to warn others of significant dangers.
3. *Specifiable Duty of General Beneficence.* All individuals have a general obligation to help others (an obligation of general beneficence), the contours of which are not clear in advance but are subject to specification in ways that depend on individuals' circumstances.

The only one of these assumptions that is new to our discussion so far is the specifiable duty of beneficence. The importance of the rights of privacy, as I argued in the previous chapter, is presumed by our practice of obtaining informed consent. I shall have more to say, below, in defense of the claim that we actually have such privacy rights; however, I expect that many of my readers will be willing to take this for granted. The duty to warn is a special case of the duty of rescue, also encountered in the previous chapter. I do take for granted that we have general obligations of beneficence that go beyond the duty of (easy) rescue. In common with many, I assume that the demandingness of our beneficence obligations is contextually variable, being sensitive to such matters as the sort of relationship one has with the person needing help. Our duties to help, I assume, are demanding but differentiated in myriad ways. Friendship, family relations, and even a shared history

60

of joint activity can provide a basis for specially demanding duties of beneficence directed to particular persons (see, e.g., Kolodny, 2010). These various, conventionally shaped networks of activity and relationship can shape and specify our duties of beneficence, which are otherwise rather amorphous. I further assume that moral theory should for many purposes take many of our conventions as given, while always holding open the possibility of criticizing them.[2] This book, for instance, takes as given the fact that our practices recognize as a distinct occupation that of a scientist doing medical research involving human subjects.

Against the background of these assumptions, my explanation of the special ancillary-care obligation, in a nutshell, is as follows (Fig. 2): Subjects' privacy rights (1) are selectively waived during the informed-consent process (4). This waiver is not *purely* permission-giving, but also results in (5) some transfer of responsibility. When an ancillary-care need is discovered (6), this special responsibility would generate a duty of tactful silence (7), except that this is blocked by (2) the duty to warn; it hence generates instead (8) a duty of tactful engagement that provides the needed sort of circumstantial focus for (3) the specifiable duty of beneficence, resulting in a special ancillary-care obligation (9).

Which responsibilities get transferred when rights are waived? As I will argue below, the ones tied to the core function of the rights being waived. The core function of the relevant privacy rights, I will suggest, is to provide control over access to certain facts so as to help shield fragile aspects of individuals' autonomy. To have special responsibilities about such matters means having special obligations of *tactfulness* towards their research participants. Often, tact in relation to sensitive subjects requires that one remain silent

---

2. I develop my views on the relationships among convention, moral objectivity, and moral theory in Richardson (forthcoming).

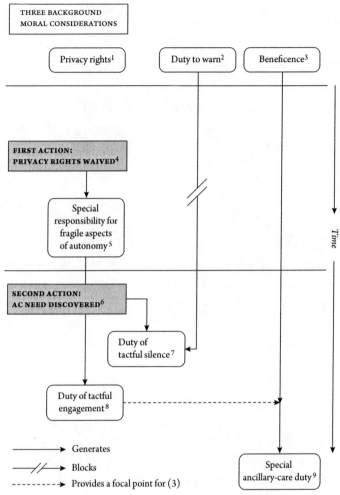

Figure 2. The Elements Generating Privacy-Based Moral Entanglements

about them. When, however, a researcher has discovered a significant ancillary-care need of which the participant is unaware, the
duty to warn blocks the option of silence. In those cases, then, tact
instead requires treating the person with special care. This provides a special focus for the specifiable duty of general beneficence

that lies in the background, giving rise to a special ancillary-care obligation.

In developing this account, this chapter will range quite widely over other professions aside from that of medical research and, significantly, over cases that do not involve any kind of professional interaction. If this account is sound, then it implies that the special ancillary-care obligation is not essentially an obligation of a professional towards a client. The account does tie the scope of the obligation to the obtaining of special permissions that, in our society, marks the inception of a professional relationship between medical researchers and their research participants; but the present chapter's account of the grounds of this special obligation indicates that it is the acceptance of these permissions that does the moral work and not the existence of a professional relationship as such. On this matter, the approach I defend here departs from the way that Miller, Mello, and Joffe (2008) develop the idea of partial entrustment. In addressing in Chapter 7 the implications of our accounts for the question of incidental findings—their focus in that article—I will draw out the practical implications of this difference in conceptual approach.

One challenge that any such account of the grounds of partial entrustment must meet, as I have mentioned, is to explain why the scope of entrustment is limited in the way the theory suggests. The scope limitation, as I interpret it, is based on the informational route whereby the researchers become aware of the need for care. Because the account I will develop in this chapter focuses on rights to privacy concerning one's body and medical history, it gives the relevant information a central place. Accordingly, it will provide the needed explanation of the scope limitation.

It will also help the partial-entrustment model meet a second, equally important challenge. We have seen that clinical medical research, to be ethically permissible, should be socially valuable.

Often, though certainly not always, medical research holds out the prospect of benefiting either the individual participants or the community of which they are a part. The malaria researchers in the Malaria Researchers and Schistosomiasis case, for instance, are presumably doing their part in a broader global effort to find ways to help reduce the suffering that malaria imposes on communities such as the one in which they are working. In this way, these researchers are already being quite helpful to these communities. Further, in providing even fairly basic care for malaria, as part of even the minimally acceptable "standard of care" for such studies, they are also benefiting the individual participants. Imagine that these researchers are medical doctors from the United States. They might have chosen to do bench research back at home or to have worked as infectious-disease clinicians in the safer and more comfortable environment of a U.S. hospital. Instead, they have decided to work in difficult conditions on the front lines of the war against malaria. Without presuming anything in particular about their underlying motivations, still we can say that these doctors have undertaken some real personal burden in order to help those suffering from malaria. Why, then, is it reasonable to suppose that, by undertaking their malaria research, they take on an *additional*, special obligation of care? We may call this the "burdening-the-helper" objection.[3]

To address the burdening-the-helper objection, I will make a point, in this chapter, of looking around more broadly. Medical

3. Alan Wertheimer raised this objection in discussions of these issues, and has now articulated it in print (Wertheimer, 2011, 257, 283). As he points out (313), this incredulity about the greater claims of the already benefited is closely related to what Samuel Scheffler (2001, 56–57) called the "distributive objection," which raises doubts about how a relationship between two parties could properly be taken to redound to the moral disadvantage of a third. Note, however, that, on my account, the basis of special claims rests on an actual history of transaction, and thus, contrary to what Wertheimer suggests (2011, 283), does not come into play when comparing two hypothetical cases.

researchers' special ancillary-care obligations, I will suggest, are instances of a moral phenomenon we encounter more broadly in everyday life, albeit not one that philosophers have paid much attention to. This phenomenon, which I will "moral entanglement," is one whereby special obligations unintendedly arise in a way that is ancillary to some other moral transaction. There are many paths by which we can stumble into special moral obligations in an unplanned and unintended way, getting morally entangled without doing any wrong. Most simply and familiarly, this will happen in the course of forming "a relationship" with someone.[4] Yet cases of consent-based moral entanglements arising out of waivers of privacy rights are also relatively easy to find once you go looking for them. Here, I seek both to begin to map out the broader category of privacy-based moral entanglements and to mount a defense of the claim that privacy-based moral entanglements really exist: that we really can take on unintended and even unforeseen special obligations by accepting another's waiver of privacy rights. What gives rise to the new obligation in which the entanglement consists? My claim will be that it is the shift in the parties' moral statuses—in their claims and obligations constituted by the acceptance of the privacy waiver—and not merely some shift in the causal possibilities consequent upon this change in the parties' moral statuses. At the end of the chapter, I will take up opponents who instead focus more impartially (more "agent-neutrally," as philosophers would put it) on these causal shifts.

The sort of privacy-based moral entanglement I have in mind can arise in everyday life, outside the context of any professional

---

4. Hence, I do not deny that, by becoming friendly with the waitresses at the café where they have lunch every day, medical researchers might gain some special obligation to help these waitresses. What I deny, rather, is that they would gain this special obligation *as* researchers (cf. Richardson, 2009).

context, when someone is just being helpful. The following case illustrates how:

> *The Old Man and the Groceries:* You see an old man, a stranger to you, struggling to carry a bag of groceries that is clearly too heavy for him. Finding out that he lives around the corner from you, you offer to carry them, and he accepts. On the way home, you find out that he lives alone. At his front door, there is some delay as he fumbles with his keys due to his obviously quite severely limited eyesight. Once you're inside and have deposited the bag on the kitchen table, you see that the kitchen counters and sink are piled high with scraps of rotten food, all growing dangerous-looking colonies of mold that, apparently, he cannot see or smell. Should you help him clean up this mess?

I take it that it is doubtful that any general, unspecified obligation of beneficence requires you to do so.[5] I will argue, however, that considerations pertaining to respect for privacy can indirectly ground a special obligation of beneficence in a case like this, one going beyond and supplementing what our general obligations of beneficence require.[6]

5. If you suspect that one's general duty of beneficence may already require the bag carrier to clean up the old man's kitchen mess, I invite you to shift the case by upping the costs of helping.
6. Roughly and in general, by "a special obligation," I mean one that is not incumbent on all people who are similarly situated. This characterization needs some refinement, however, for almost any consideration might be re-described as part of an agent's situation. A more precise and useful gloss of special obligations would take account of reasons that it might be impossible for certain particular agents to find themselves in certain situations. Salient among potential reasons are facts about who they are and facts about the past. Along these lines, A. John Simmons (2005, 102) has distinguished between two types of (purported) special obligations, the associative and the transactional: "Associative accounts ground our duty…in our nonvoluntary occupation of certain duty-laden social roles," such as that of a sibling or a citizen, "while Transactional

There are surely diverse sorts of moral entanglement explicable in diverse ways. For instance, relationships can morph into friendships without anyone having planned this. Here, I want to mark out a distinctive pathway of moral entanglement, involving the waiver of privacy rights, whereby some special obligations of beneficence—importantly including medical researchers' special ancillary-care obligations—arise.

Consider our ordinary understandings of the rights of privacy pertaining to facts about oneself and one's life. I say "facts," rather than "information," as I want to lay the stress on another's becoming aware of these facts, not on the downstream issue of whether the other passes them on to third parties. In all cultures of which I am aware, people take there to be some classes of such facts to which privacy rights attach: some zones of one's life that are shielded from the prying eyes of others. These zones typically include facts about one's body and bodily functions, what goes on within one's home, and one's personal finances. Like all complex social practices, those that set the boundaries of these expectations of privacy stand in need of normative critique. Feminist philosophers, in particular, have subjected conventional ideas about privacy rights to criticism based on their potential for shielding patriarchal abuse and for perpetuating oppressive ideas about the body (e.g., MacKinnon, 1989; Nussbaum, 2004). While these critiques show the need for various reforms to our laws and our attitudes, I will assume that some privacy rights pertaining to the zones I have mentioned will remain morally justified (cf. Allen, 1988). I will argue that when one accepts another's waiver of such privacy rights—whether explicitly or, as in

accounts ground our duty (or obligation)…in our morally significant interactions" with others. In this chapter, I will be developing an account of an unfamiliar, non-contractual sort of transactional obligation that arises from the acceptance of privacy waivers. While my account of why there can be such special obligations will appeal to broader considerations, that appeal will not cancel the transactional basis of individual cases of such obligation.

The Old Man and the Groceries, implicitly—one accrues special responsibilities towards that other that can become the basis of a special obligation of beneficence.[7]

Let me explain a little more fully the sort of privacy-based moral entanglements that is worth paying attention to, here, laying down a little more terminology as I do so. Privacy rights of the kind at issue can of course be waived unilaterally. As the cases of a streaker or of someone who blurts out his or her intimate secrets to strangers on a subway car make vivid, behaviors that effect unilateral privacy waivers can themselves constitute criticizable impositions on others. Cases in which one has a choice whether to take up or accept the privacy waiver, whether explicitly or by some action such as entering the other's home, are quite different. The case of medical researchers is such a case, one in which the voluntariness that attaches to accepting the privacy waivers is usually expressed in the researchers having *solicited* the privacy waivers through the informed-consent process. It is the mutually voluntary type of case on which I focus. After a bilaterally voluntary process of offer and acceptance or proffer and uptake, people agree that the privacy rights of one of them be relaxed. That gives the other access to zones those privacy rights normally protect, such as their bodies, their homes, or their financial records; they have, I will say, created "intimacies." These intimacies constitute morally defined relationships that may be deep or limited, standing or ad hoc, and of varying degrees of intimacy.

People enter into intimacies, so defined, for highly various reasons. Sometimes people establish intimacies simply in order to share a secret with someone else, typically saddling their confidants with confidentiality obligations. Those intimacies do not concern me here. Instead, I will be focusing on intimacies that arise when

7. My claim is limited to cases in which the waiver of privacy rights actually results in access to private matters. Throughout, I will assume that the privacy waivers are taken up or accepted so that such access is gained.

people waive their privacy rights for other reasons, such as to obtain medical treatment or legal advice or to have sex with someone. These other reasons provide the principal purpose for the interaction, the moral entanglements that arise being incidental and unintended. Of course, confidentiality obligations may arise in some of these cases, too. Confidentiality obligations do not require one to do anything on the basis of the information, only to safeguard it. Important as confidentiality obligations are in the context of medical research, these are not the obligations that matter for our understanding of ancillary-care obligations. Here, in an attempt to explicate these, I will concentrate instead on a less familiar class of obligations (or wrong-making considerations) arising from intimacies, ones that require one not merely to process what one has learned from having been given access to the private but also to act on it in a way that exercises a broader range and heightened level of care (compared to baseline) towards the person who shared it. Those who agree to be someone's confidant should perhaps know to expect such duties of follow-up; but those who have accepted privacy waivers implicitly or explicitly offered by a person seeking medical treatment, legal proceedings, sex, or even a stranger's help, will generally not have expected or intended to become anyone's confidant. And even without becoming a confidant, they may, to their surprise, find themselves morally entangled via what they learn by acting on the privacy waivers. Among the resulting obligations will be some that are not only not planned or intended results of the interaction but also quite ancillary to their purposes in interacting. That is, they are "ancillary-care obligations" of a generic kind (not specifically tied to medical research).[8] I will concentrate on explaining how intimacies

8. In Richardson & Belsky (2004) and Belsky & Richardson (2004), we defined "ancillary care" more narrowly, in a way that perhaps overly anticipated our conclusion that ancillary-care obligations cannot be reduced to other, more familiar sorts of obligations applicable in that context. In the present chapter, I use "ancillary care" more broadly,

can give rise to moral entanglements and, specifically, to ancillary-care obligations of this generic kind.

To move in the direction of such an account, I will need to begin with a brief survey of the relevant moral phenomena, classifying entangling intimacies and indicating what a lot of them have in common. Not infrequently, someone who has been given access to private matters finds therein dangers or concerns of which the person whose matters they are is apparently unaware. Accordingly, at the threshold of ancillary duties of care often lies a duty to warn. I will take this threshold issue up next, focusing on potential moral inhibitions on warning and how these interact with the acceptance of privacy waivers. Because, as I will argue, the creation of intimacies tends to cancel moral inhibitions on the duty to warn, one generally may not evade intimacy-based moral entanglements by remaining mum about serious problems one discovers via the access one obtains by accepting waivers of privacy. Once having confirmed that this escape route is out of the way, I will turn to the positive argument that special ancillary-care obligations, which require more effort than a simple warning, arise from intimacies. Because, as I have indicated, this argument turns on the fact that accepting rights waivers gives one special responsibility for the considerations underlying the relevant rights, I will first lay out some of those considerations. My aim ultimately will be to show that given that the duty to warn constrains one to put the difficulty on the table, one's accrued special responsibility for these considerations underlying privacy rights in turn supports a special duty of beneficence focused on the need that is now out in the open between the two parties (see again Fig. 2, above). Before closing the chapter, I will consider whether a non-transactional view could provide a satisfactory account of this territory.

---

concentrating on articulating the specific kind of moral entanglement that explains how there can be special ancillary-care obligations.

## A RANGE OF INTIMACIES

As I have said, I think that medical researchers' special ancillary-care obligations are an instance of a kind of moral entanglement that, while quite common, is not well understood. To grasp the nature of this obligation, we need to survey the terrain of privacy-based moral entanglements more generally. In thinking about the range of intimacies that we encounter, it is useful to recognize that the point of the interaction can vary considerably. Sometimes the point is to get some help. In a paradigm such case, which we might call a "helping intimacy," one person waives privacy rights as a means to obtaining help and the other accepts that waiver in order to provide it. Any other case we may call a "non-helping intimacy." Of course, people entering a helping intimacy might have done so for all sorts of ulterior reasons. Personal physicians and tax accountants, for instance, need to accept privacy waivers as a means to exercising their professions and thereby earning a living; but they each earn a living *by* helpfully processing private information. The notion of "helping" that I am invoking here is neither unfamiliar nor unproblematic. It is found in the rather smug and self-congratulatory self-description of the professions of clinical medicine, nursing, and psychotherapy as "helping professions." As opposed to car mechanics and cooks, who hurt people?[9] No. The relevant notion of helping does not contrast principally either with selfish behavior or with behavior that is obligatory. My point in distinguishing the helping intimacies from non-helping ones is simply to separate out the cases in which some special duty of care or of helping is already grounded in the relationship from the cases in which this is not so.

9. See the discussion thread begun by Robin Hanson in 2006 at http://www.overcoming-bias.com/2006/12/do_helping_prof.html (accessed 8/25/2009).

In helping intimacies, where the point of the interaction builds in or supports some focused duty of care, the entanglements we are interested in involve duties of care that are ancillary—that is, subordinate and supplementary—to the duties at the relationship's core. Describing uncontestable cases of this kind would require having in hand clear accounts of the ethics of various professions and stations of life; still, even without such a basis, we can make a start. Accountants, for instance, profess fairly high standards of professional integrity, but these are attached to relatively narrow definitions of the accountant's role. Tax fraud must be avoided and assets and liabilities must be properly balanced; but what about:

> *The Tax Accountant and the Gambling Addict:* In going over a client's statements for purposes of helping prepare the client's tax returns, an accountant notices a telltale pattern of repeated, large liquidations of stocks and bonds followed closely by equivalently large payments to Foxwoods Casino. Does the accountant have an obligation to have a serious talk with the client about the client's gambling addiction?

I take it that the accountant does have an ancillary-care responsibility, here.[10] The point of any such intervention, I take it, would

---

10. Throughout this chapter, my discussion is focused on the issue that the partial-entrustment model labels the issue of the "scope" of the special ancillary-care obligation: I am here trying to explain the general nature of this obligation. Later chapters will return to exploring its concrete implications. Now, even confining oneself to the considerations incorporated into the partial-entrustment model, items that are within the scope may fail to give rise to an actual duty because—in the extended sense captured by the "strength" test—acting on the responsibility in the given circumstances is too costly. The accountant's intruding on the client's choices about how to use his money is clearly one relevant cost, parallel to the young man's intruding on the kitchen habits of the Old Man. If these costs seem to you to be negating any duty in this case, please imagine that the financial implications of the stock liquidations that the accountant detects are quite disastrous for the client: that he is constantly being forced to sell low, for instance. I am grateful to Frank Miller for discussion of this issue.

go beyond mere warning. Its purpose would not be principally to provide information, but to modify behavior. After all, the client already knows how he has moved his money. Any such duty to try to help the client with the gambling addiction seems ancillary to the duties of care supported by the point of this kind of helping (i.e., service) relationship.

Impromptu helpers, too, can get morally entangled via privacy waivers: recall the case of The Old Man and the Groceries. One thing thus leads to another. The tax accountant and the old man's helper had each undertaken to help another. Moral entanglements, however, can also arise from non-helping intimacies.

Consider reporters and their sources. Reporters need information, often private information, and in seeking it out do not generally purport to offer any help to their potential sources. Indeed, as a matter of professional ethics, journalists are often discouraged from intervening in the lives of people they write about.[11] This is sometimes thought of as helping to ensure impartiality. It also serves as a consideration that might conflict with an entanglement such as:

*The Reporter and the Peasant:* Reporting on the likely impact of a planned hydroelectric dam on the upper Mekong, a U.S.-based reporter learns from interviewing a Laotian peasant that the peasant is apparently unaware not only of the planned dam but also of the economic ruin that awaits him if he does

---

11. In the *New York Times Magazine* of August 23, 2009, Dexter Filkins wrote as follows about his reaction to the huge email response he had received to an earlier front-page story about an Iraqi girl who had had acid thrown onto her face because she was attending school: "Journalists are not supposed to become involved with the people they write about. That's one of the craft's tenets. I have occasionally given some money to one or another of the more luckless people I've interviewed—a widow whose husband was killed by a death squad in Baghdad, for instance. But mostly I've kept my distance. This time, I decided to set the rules aside." http://www.nytimes.com/2009/08/23/magazine/23school-t.html?_r=2&pagewanted=3&sq=filkins%20afghanistan%20women&st=cse&scp=1 (accessed 8/30/2009).

not quickly get relocation help. Should the reporter tell him about the project and take an afternoon back in the provincial capital to make sure that the peasant gets onto the relocation authority's rolls?

Non-helping intimacies can also arise independently of any professional role. I will take a case involving sexual intimacy. There are risks in so doing, as sex is complicated; but it also is a context in which privacy—both as to the body and as to one's proclivities—is typically mutually waived, often without any helping purpose or intention and sometimes with the parties each simply seeking pleasure above all. Consider such a case:

> *Welts:* During a casual, mutually selfish sexual encounter, you notice that your partner's back is covered with bruises and welts. Someone is beating her. Should you try to find out about the abusive relationship she is apparently in and help extricate her from it?

In this case, as in all of my others so far, it seems to me that there is some significant moral entanglement.

In this quick survey of moral entanglements, we have seen how such unintended obligations might arise both for professionals carrying out their professional roles and for people who encounter one another casually. Crosscutting that difference, as we have also seen, they can arise for people whose role, casual or professional, is focused in a specific way on helping the other person and for people who had no helping role, professional or otherwise. The private information that appears to trigger these entanglements has been quite various: pertaining to the body, bodily or mental health, or finances. While the theory of intimacy-based moral entanglements that I shall offer will support the conclusion that there is an ancillary-care obligation in each of the cases I have presented so far, I do not mean to rest my argument principally on the cases. These I set out more with an eye to orienting the reader to this philosophically little-explored terrain. To make a convincing case that there really are such obligations, we need a plausible theory of how moral entanglements arise out of intimacies. Since they seem to arise in a context rich with other obligations, an important part of the theoretical task will be to keep track of the distinct contributions of these various other factors. One such factor, which looks like it might explain much that lies in the vicinity of moral entanglements, is the duty to warn.

## THE DUTY TO WARN

In this discussion of moral entanglements, the duty to warn plays a halfway-house role in more ways than one. Warning the other is a potentially useful response in many of my cases because, rather than sharing a loaded secret with you, the other has permitted you access to private information from which you have concluded that there is a problem. Because warning someone is typically so easy, a duty to warn can usually be seen as instantiating the *general* duty of rescue. The duty of rescue (as articulated, for instance, in Scanlon's Rescue Principle, quoted in the previous chapter) is general in the sense that it directs one to help another independently of any past transaction or association between the two people. The duty of rescue reflects an important alternative to moral entanglement, one that might explain many cases without calling upon any special duties or obligations and without distinguishing among different ways one person has learned about the danger another faces. Hence, at one level, the duty of rescue competes with the idea of moral entanglements in explaining the moral appearances. One possible way of resisting this competing explanation would be to deny the existence of a general duty of rescue. Compelling defenses of the duty of rescue have been offered, however (e.g., McIntyre, 1994; Scanlon, 1998). Accordingly, I will not take that route. I see special ancillary-care obligations—both generically and in the special case of those attaching to medical research—as supplementing the general duty of rescue rather than competing with it. Accordingly, I will argue that, in many areas of life, duties of ancillary care can go beyond what would be called for by the duty of rescue.

My account of the grounds of these special ancillary-care obligations will *rely* on there also being a duty to warn in these cases. Examining how privacy waivers can remove moral inhibitions on warning will be helpful to my account. The moral inhibitions on warning may be ranged under the heading of "minding your own business." There are always reasons to tread carefully when responding to private information. There is the danger that one will do no good and simply upset the person. There is also the danger of being paternalistically judgmental about another's lifestyle (cf. O'Neill, 1985).[12] Perhaps the old man likes living in a kitchen redolent of previous meals and is happy to give his immune system exercise; perhaps what looks like a gambling addiction from the tax accountant's point of view is simply the client's number-one priority in life.

It seems to be fairly widely accepted that there are some moral inhibitions on a doctor warning a stranger at a bus stop about a suspicious-looking mole (Zwitter et al., 1999, 252; cf. Moseley, 1985, and Ratzen, 1985). Whatever the exact nature of the moral inhibitions on a doctor's warning a stranger on the street, they are erased by the formation of a doctor–patient or researcher–participant relationship. There may be many reasons for this difference,

---

12. I am grateful to Adrienne Martin for reminding me of this classic article and to Victoria McGeer for pointing out the danger of paternalism.

however. In the case of clinicians, for instance, it may be that doctors' "Hippocratic" role responsibility to look after the patient's health is here the overwhelming reason why there is no such moral inhibition (cf. Pellegrino, 2001). To come closer to isolating the difference that the acceptance of privacy waivers might make, let us temporarily steer away from the core "helping profession" of medicine and think, instead, about:

> *The Massage Therapist and the Mole:* From his years dealing with skin, the massage therapist has come to have a very good eye for dangerous moles.
>
> *Variant I:* While he is waiting in the corridor of the health club for his next client to get ready, another patron—as it happens another regular massage client, this day in the gym for another reason—comes out of the locker room on the way to the steam room, slips on the wet floor and almost falls, meanwhile letting go of the towel around his waist, allowing the massage therapist (who has glanced up involuntarily to make sure he is OK) clearly to see for the first time a dangerous-looking mole on his buttocks.
>
> *Variant II:* While, at the client's request, working out a knot in the client's glutes, the massage therapist notices a dangerous-looking mole on the client's buttocks.

It seems to me that there are some significant moral inhibitions against warning in Variant I that are not present in Variant II. My suggestion, of course, is that in the latter case, these moral inhibitions are largely cancelled by the implicit but fully accepted waiver of bodily privacy. This waiver is narrowly contextual and does not cover cases off of the massage table in which one might accidentally expose one's flesh (as in Variant I). Intuitively, it seems that the acceptance of a privacy waiver in Variant II makes the mole the massage therapist's "business" in a way that it is not in Variant I. In this way, the acceptance of privacy waivers can overcome a potential defeasor of the duty to warn. Note that in both variants there is the same basic masseur–client relationship between the two people involved; the difference to which I am pointing does not have to do with the general relationship but with its particular transactional history.

We began this section with the thought that the general duty of rescue is a possible competitor to the idea of special moral entanglements. We then took a closer look at a special case of rescue, the duty to warn. This seemed to reveal that waivers of privacy, which are crucial to building some entanglements, also modulate the duty to warn. This is encouraging, for it suggests that the duty to warn is not clearly in opposition to them and may in fact be sensitive to the same sort of moral considerations that these entanglements involve. With this conclusion in hand, I will now turn to privacy-based entanglements proper. In fact, as I have signaled, my account of these entanglements will build on the duty to warn. Since my account of this specific range of entanglements draws on some of the considerations underlying the relevant privacy rights, I will first expound these. My claim will eventually be that in the context of intimacies in which a duty to warn arises, these considerations switch from being reasons to keep one's distance to reasons why one ought to help.

## AUTONOMY-CENTERED REASONS
## FOR PRIVACY RIGHTS

There are no doubt many important moral considerations that go towards supporting privacy rights of the kind I am focusing on here, which are overrideable, directed claims that pertain to zones such as one's body, one's home, and one's financial records.[13] Judith Wagner DeCew (2006) has recently catalogued some of the considerations that have been put forward: "control over information about oneself," "human dignity," enabling of "intimacy" or "meaningful interpersonal relationships," and "[enhancement of] personal expression and choice." Were the task to account, generally, for the moral importance of privacy rights, my tendency would be to support DeCew in her view that some broad combination of these considerations is needed to explain the moral importance of the kinds of privacy rights we are discussing (DeCew, 1997). In this section, thankfully, my task is different: I aim simply to single out in a way that will be relevant to medical research a pervasively important subset of the considerations that back up privacy rights. These considerations have to do with a relatively deep way in which control over information about oneself supports personal expression and choice. These last two factors of course can be connected in a relatively shallow and obvious way: By enhancing individuals' control over the release and spreading of information about themselves, privacy rights can help shield a person's expressions and choices from criticism and reprisal, and so from various costs and unpleasantness.

There is, however, also a deeper way of linking these factors of control and personal choice. It involves the idea of autonomy, by which I here mean to refer to the kind of personal capacities involved in being a self-governing agent. The connecting thought is that some important type of control over information about oneself is crucial to supporting one's capacity to be an autonomous agent, and hence to be able to exercise "personal choice" in any robust sense. Admittedly, this statement is quite vague. I have no intention

---

13. On the nature of overrideable, directed claims, which correlate with duties owed to particular people, see Sreenivasan (2010).

of trying here to sharpen up the idea of autonomy sufficiently for us to assess whether some control over personal information is a necessary condition of autonomy. Instead, we may simply identify some contingent supports for autonomy that can vary by degrees and whose total absence would at least be a great blow to autonomy, which can be more or less robust. (The idea that autonomy requires contingent support is, at one level, an un-Kantian thought, one that we should accept as an important correction to Kant: cf. Honneth, 1995.) Paul Benson (1994) has well described one such support for autonomy: one's sense of one's own competence in executing one's actions in a way that can, in the ways that one hopes and expects, minimally live up to the expectations of others. Explicating this notion, he adduced the vivid example of the movie "Gaslight," in which the wife (Ingrid Bergman) is so worked upon by her evil husband (Charles Boyer) that she comes to lose all confidence in her ability to carry out even the simplest sorts of action in any social setting. Here, I would like to highlight another aspect of agential self-confidence, one concerned not with one's ability to execute one's plans and aims but with one's ability to frame one's aims—to make up one's mind—in the first place.

I am not talking about what Diana Tietjens Meyers calls the "androcentric phantasm" of a transparent and unitary self that makes up its own mind in "unfettered independence from other individuals." As she notes, while feminist theorists have rightly criticized extreme, individualistic versions of autonomy, they seem largely to have come to accept the importance of being able to govern oneself in the ways this may be done by a complex self immersed in many kinds of relationships with others (Meyers, 2000, 152). It is autonomy understood in the latter way that I have in mind.

In explaining how confidence in one's ability to make up one's own mind depends on privacy, let me start with the familiar case of parents and children. Fostering a child's capacity to make up his or her own mind about things is one of a parent's most uncomfortable and important tasks. As Tamar Schapiro (1999, 736) has written, "our end as adults cannot be to control children; it must be to make them free to control themselves." Parents must step back and allow children to make their own mistakes, even ones involving injury and pain. Initially, children are allowed simply some scope for freedom of action, but eventually they must be allowed to form their own plans and to attempt to "discover" themselves, even by parents who think they understand their children better than they yet understand themselves. In articulating these commonplace thoughts, the language of "allowing" the children to make their own decisions comes naturally; but this allowing should not be conflated with merely giving permission. Yes, parents must permit children scope for free action; but, beyond that, they must communicate to their children that they can and must make up their own minds without constantly checking back to see what their parents expect or whether they are meeting those expectations. And parents cannot communicate this truly or convincingly unless they allow their children some privacy in forming and carrying out their plans. Hence, fostering a child's capacity for autonomous action importantly requires parents to respect their children's privacy in a significant way.

Excessively tight parental control is simply the most accessible example of a threat to a healthy and confident capacity to make up one's own mind. Maintaining this capacity can be a life-long struggle. A few decades back, philosophical discussions of personal autonomy were more focused on another such case, that of so-called "oppressive socialization" (e.g., Christman, 1986 and 2001; Benson 1991). We do not need a theory of oppression, here, to remind us that it is not only parents whose attentions can be suffocating and can choke out room adequately to develop the capacity to frame one's own aims: the label, "oppression," suffices. Peers, teachers, religious institutions, and broad cultural practices can each have a hand in stifling or undoing this development. Nor should the nurturing of this ability in the transition from childhood to adulthood be our only concern, for in a sufficiently oppressive environment, even people who have well developed the ability to make up their own minds may largely lose it, and fall into abject dependence, reflexive deference, or practical paralysis. Privacy rights are needed to shield individuals from the attentions and appraisals by these persons, institutions, and broad cultural groups, thus protecting individuals' capacity to frame their aims.

Yet it is also obvious that we cannot and should not shield people from all attention from and appraisal by their parents, peers, teachers, religious communities, or culture more broadly. For one thing, much of the socializing influence from each of these sources is not merely benign but actually valuable and can often support autonomy. For another, we need to watch and sanction people so that they do not harm others. Hence, it makes sense that the privacy rights supported by this kind of concern for autonomy do not simply shield anyone in a blanket way from the attentions of others. Instead, our privacy rights are connected to this concern somewhat indirectly, by being attached to zones in which the concern is particularly salient.[14] Here, for illustrative purposes, I have focused on three zones: one's body, one's personal finances, and one's home. While each might saliently connect with people's fragile capacity to make up their own minds in various ways, here are a couple of suggestions about the most important such connections. From the point of view of protecting individuals' capacity to frame their aims, the case for shielding their bodies and their personal finances

14. What I am offering, here, is a rational reconstruction of how the zones of privacy we are familiar with in our everyday practices subserve the aspect of autonomy I have focused on, not anything remotely like an historical account of how these privacy expectations arose.

from unwanted attentions can rest on the fact that these are highly sensitive areas. They tend to be the focus of insecurities that make us highly reactive to expressed approval or disapproval by others. I take it that this is obvious enough in the case of the body, given how insecure it can make us to feel ugly or deformed or ill. The case of The Tax Accountant and the Gambling Addict illustrates how vulnerability to criticism—as well as the shallower dimension of vulnerability to reprisal and manipulation—can arise in one's personal finances. Privacy with regard to one's home or residence supports one's capacity to frame one's aims in a different way. It shields a space in which one can try out and express one's practical conception of who one is, whether by playing air guitar in the living room or by decorating one's den in a way that expresses one's fantasies about being a jungle explorer.

So: given our social practices, individuals have privacy rights regarding their bodies, their homes, and their personal finances, among other things. I take it that we reflectively endorse these social practices, at least in outline, doubtless for many reasons. In this section, my aim has simply been to point to one important reason why such privacy rights should be accorded, namely that they are crucial to supporting individuals' capacities to frame and select their own aims, enabling them to develop and express those capacities without fear. These capacities, like more executive forms of agential self-confidence, are, in turn, crucial supports of autonomy. This link between privacy rights and autonomy is a contingent and empirical one, not a conceptual one, but an important one for all that. In societies with radically different conventions and practices, privacy rights might well focus on different zones; but it is hard to imagine their not being justified in a similar way. In what follows, I will assume that a threat to this sort of agential self-confidence is a threat to autonomy. In the next section, I will argue that the relations between promoting and respecting the other's autonomy are complicated by accepting another's waiver of such a privacy right. A closer look at these complications will reveal an argument for the kind of ancillary-care duties that arise in privacy-based moral entanglements, including those linking medical researchers to their research participants.

## ANCILLARY DUTIES OF CARE

I am now in a position to explain how special, ancillary duties of care arise from privacy waivers. My claim is that by voluntarily entering into an intimacy one takes on some broad responsibilities related to the grounds of the privacy rights that were waived in its formation and that, depending on how things go, these responsibilities can give rise to special ancillary-care obligations. These will extend to helping the other deal with a problem that one has discovered via the intimacy, warned the other about, and been asked by the other to help with.

The resulting ancillary-care obligations are thus special obligations, for they thoroughly depend on the transactions that have occurred between the relevant individuals. To explain these transactions clearly, while maintaining a general focus that takes in not only medical research but also other contexts in which privacy-based moral entanglements arise, I will need a little more terminology. While this terminology may sound fussily legalistic, its point is just to help us keep track of who is who. Thus, we need to distinguish between the one who proffered the privacy waiver (the "offeror") and the one who accepted it (the "accepter").[15] Using

15. Throughout the present chapter, I will assume that the person who accepts the privacy waiver is also the person who gets the access to private information that this waiver permits. In other words, I will ignore cases in which the accepter is serving as the agent of someone else, on whose behalf the privacy waiver is sought or accepted. This

this terminology, we may return to the three relevant aspects of the transactions between these two individuals mentioned in the previous paragraph. There is the basic fact that has set up the intimacy, namely that the privacy waiver that gave rise to it was mutually voluntary. Then there are two additional key facts about how the interaction between these two should or might unfold further, involving warnings and requests for help. In cases involving the accepter's discovery of a significant ancillary need in the offeror, of which the offeror seems to be unaware, the accepter incurs a duty to warn and hence should proceed to offer a warning. I will confine my argument to such cases, which include the paradigmatic cases of medical researchers' ancillary-care obligations. As I argued earlier in this chapter, the privacy waiver sidelines some of the normal moral inhibitions on warning. Once having warned the other, the accepter should (as I will argue in a moment) give the offeror a chance to ask for help. If the offeror does not ask for help, the accepter should probably back off; but if the offeror asks for help (or indicates that he or she would like help), then the accepter comes under a special obligation to provide it. The initial, mutually voluntary establishment of a privacy waiver—often a one-sided one—sets up a basic voluntary assumption of responsibility, one that potentially makes certain vulnerabilities of the offeror of special moral concern to the accepter. The later facts about how the interaction unfolds brings to light one of these vulnerabilities, generating a reason why the background obligation of beneficence specially applies.

That's the picture, then: Against the assumed backdrop of privacy rights, a duty to warn, and a contextually specifiable general duty of beneficence, an accepted waiver of privacy rights sets the stage for a special duty of ancillary care, should some relevant

---

question of agency will arise, though, in Chapter 7, in connection with research done on samples in biobanks.

need come to light, by transferring certain responsibilities to the accepter. I have diagrammed this view above, with emphasis on its moral elements (see Fig. 2). Now I am finally in a position to justify the view. In doing so, I will attend especially to the connections among these elements (Fig. 3).

The crucial connections are the following ones:

A. How accepting the offeror's waiver of privacy rights transfers to the accepter's special responsibility for fragile aspects of the offeror's autonomy

B. How the duty to warn blocks fulfilling that special responsibility by maintaining a tactful silence

C. How the duty to warn thus shifts the practical implications of this special responsibility towards a duty of tactful engagement

D. How the duty of tactful engagement provides a focus for the specifiable duty of general beneficence

I will begin by explaining how accepting privacy waivers involves a special assumption of responsibility.

## Why Those Accepting Privacy Waivers Take on Special Responsibilities

Waivers of rights serve, by definition, to confer permissions; but they often do more than that. We are familiar in everyday life with how accepting another's waiver of rights involves a shift in the default allocation of moral responsibility. Or perhaps the way to put it is that in everyday life, we simply do not often encounter *pure* waivers of rights—transactions whose moral effect is limited to a permission-giving. We saw this at the outset with privacy waivers, for we saw that waivers of privacy often come coupled with the establishment

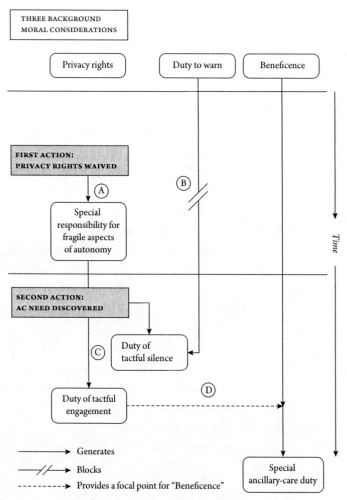

Figure 3. Privacy-Based Moral Entanglements: Putting the Pieces Together

of special responsibilities or obligations to see to it that the confidentiality of the private information in question is well safeguarded. It is one and the same transaction that both waives the right and gives rise to this responsibility. How so? I suggest we see the waiver, in these situations, as part of a broader alienation of the right in question in which responsibilities of the erstwhile right-holder attaching to the right get transferred or delegated to the accepter.

Arguing first by analogy, I will first illustrate this point about alienation with an example before trying to explain it more generally.[16] If your friend waives his right to the exclusive use of his car and lets you borrow it, then—without any explicit agreement between the two of you—you take on some of the risks that can attend driving a car, including such things as taking care of dealing with any dents or scrapes that appeared when you left it in some parking lot or arranging for a jump start if the battery runs dead while you had the car parked somewhere.[17] These responsibilities are obligations you owe to the car's owner, in contrast to the general obligation you have to operate the vehicle with due care for the welfare of pedestrians and other drivers. The right to exclusive use of the car gives its owner some degree of control over risks of damage and malfunction and over how to deal with them if they arise. By accepting the owner's waiver of this right, you take on some moral responsibility for such risks, should they crop up during your use of the car, even when this is no fault of yours. Some of the ill moral luck associated with the car now falls your direction. This will be so whether or not these risks occurred to you at the time you accepted the use of the car. Perhaps it is revealing that we do not ask our friends whether they will waive their right to exclusive use of their vehicles; we ask

16. The car-borrowing example I give in this paragraph is one that typically involves someone soliciting the waiver of a right as a necessary step to obtaining a favor from the rightholder. In that respect, the case has more in common with the Malaria Researchers and Schistosomiasis case than it does with The Old Man and the Groceries. Another feature of the latter case, however, is that the old man is apparently somewhat dependent on the person who helped with the groceries also to help in some way with the ancillary mess. A modification of the car-borrowing example that removed the favor-granting feature but offsettingly added this dependency feature would, I think, still serve to support the paragraph's general claim that accepting rights waivers generally modifies the distribution of responsibility.
17. I am grateful to Ezekiel Emanuel for these examples.

if we may use them. Although permission to use the vehicles is the most obvious moral change instituted by an affirmative answer, some responsibilities are simultaneously shifted to the borrower.

What is going on, here, can be analyzed in terms of the social purposes served by a system of private ownership in motor vehicles. In suggesting this, I do not mean to insist on any deep teleology; rather, I think it is fairly innocuous and non-controversial to say that private ownership in motor vehicles is not simply a plain-vanilla instance of the right of private ownership in products of manufacture. Motor vehicles, because of their portability and the dangers they pose to life and limb, to the environment, and to free passage along crowded city streets, are rightly regulated. These regulations generally attach to their ownership, requiring owners to get their vehicles insured, regularly inspected, and so on. Because of the dangers that motor vehicles pose, it is an important part of any full justification of the rights of private ownership of motor vehicles that there be a systematic way of seeing to it that these dangers are minimized. We can thus say that, given our system of the private ownership of motor vehicles, a moral responsibility falls to their owners to maintain them well and to see to it that they do not sit about, inoperable (with dead batteries, say), clogging up the streets. While the details will vary contextually, some such responsibilities seem built into, or to accompany, rights of vehicle ownership. When a vehicle's owner transfers some of those rights to you by letting you use it, it makes sense that some of these responsibilities get transferred to you with the permission. By virtue of accepting and acting upon the permission—that is, because you are using the car—you are now temporarily in a better position to look after some of these social concerns than is the owner.[18]

---

18. That you have come by these responsibilities by virtue of the permission is what crucially distinguishes my account from the "least-cost threat avoider" account to be discussed in the next section. If you have simply taken the car without permission,

The general thought, then, is that many rights come bundled with responsibilities and that many instances of what look superficially simply like acts of consent or permission-giving also involve a transfer or delegation of some of the right-holder's responsibilities to the permittee. In these instances, if you like, the permission temporarily entrusts the permittee with the carrying out of some of these responsibilities. This account of transferred responsibilities thus explains the kind of talk of "entrustment" employed by the partial-entrustment model.

Which moral responsibilities fall one's way when one voluntarily accepts someone's waiver of rights? That is, what is the scope of moral entanglements? This question is too broad to answer fully in the abstract. My general suggestion—and the answer I will carry over to the partial-entrustment model of medical researchers' special ancillary-care obligations—is that to address it we must look to the moral grounds of the right in question. Without adopting a reductively instrumentalist understanding of rights, we can recognize that rights serve moral functions in the way exemplified by the account of motor-vehicle ownership just sketched and by the last section's account of privacy rights. Moral rights institute a default division of (forward-looking) moral responsibility: the responsibility to look after one concern or another (cf. Richardson, 1999). Waivers of rights constitute a departure from that default division, shifting responsibilities by shifting rights.[19] The example of borrowing a friend's car illustrates that these responsibilities can shift in

---

you will owe the owner repairs by way of reparation for the wrong. What if, however, without having had an opportunity to ask permission, you have commandeered the car to effect an urgent rescue? In that case, it is not obvious to me whether any special responsibility to look after the vehicle's maintenance falls to you.

19. The question will arise whether those who waive their privacy rights may also waive any attendant claims to ancillary care. In Chapter 5, I argue that while research participants generally have the power to waive their claims, there are nonetheless important moral limits on what these waivers can accomplish and on the appropriateness of asking them to waive these claims.

ways not explained by any agreement but instead by reference to the functions of these rights. Instead of resting on any agreement, a post-waiver allocation of moral responsibility, I suggest, will typically be appropriately sensitive to the sort of grounds there are for the right that has been waived. The previous section gave an account of the core grounds of privacy rights of the kind relevant in medical research. Drawing on that account, we can say that what the accepter implicitly thereby takes on is a heightened responsibility for averting any threats to the offeror's autonomy or agential self-confidence that stem from sensitive private facts about the offeror coming out into the open.

## How the Duty to Warn Blocks Maintaining a Tactful Silence

Such a special responsibility readily explains how the accepter thus accrues an obligation to safeguard the confidentiality of these matters. But how can this same fact explain how intimacies give rise to ancillary-care obligations? If one has assumed heightened responsibility for shielding the other from possibly autonomy-inhibiting social disapproval, then when one encounters an unexpected problem within the other's zone of privacy as a result of a privacy waiver, one might think that what one must do is to keep a respectful distance, staying mum about it and proceeding as if one had never noticed it. Would that not be the height of the tact?[20]

Normally, yes; but in the cases of moral entanglement we have considered this is not so. In these cases, it would be morally criticizable to attempt to fulfill one's heightened responsibilities for averting threats to the offeror's autonomy or agential self-confidence by means of a tactful silence. In some of these cases, one has gleaned

---

20. I am grateful to an anonymous referee for having raised this issue of tact.

from the private facts—the mold on the old man's counters, the mole on the massage client's buttocks, the pattern of the client's casino payments, or the peasant's ignorance about the dam's impending impact—that the offeror has a fairly serious problem of which he or she is likely unaware. In those cases, the duty to warn comes into play, defeating the case for silence. (Since pursuing non-ideal theory at this fine-grained a level does not seem advisable, I will not attempt to say what should happen if the accepter fails in this duty to warn.) In the case Welts, where the apparent abuse was in the past, it is the seriousness of the wrong and its possible recurrence that calls for bringing the matter out into the open between you. In all of these cases, there are strong moral reasons to speak with the other about these facts and their significance.

## How the Duty to Warn Indirectly Supports Tactful Engagement

Bringing such facts out into the open, however, importantly reconstitutes the relationship on a new footing, making it morally criticizable to walk away: one has become morally entangled. The warning or, more generally, the broaching of the sensitive issue deepens the relationship between these two parties. Absent the warning, one had a relationship that was simply constituted as one of limited intimacy, in which a privacy right of one of the parties had been waived. Once the additional, ancillary issue has been broached, however, both parties come face-to-face with an issue with regard to which the offeror needs help. Insofar as the demandingness of beneficence obligations varies directly with the depth of relationships, this deepening of the relationship is itself a basis for firmer obligations of beneficence.

The issue is tricky, however, as this deepened intimacy also seems to be just the sort of situation that privacy rights seem designed to avoid: a situation in which the gaze of another threatens to inhibit how one deals with particularly sensitive matters. The morally required warning further heightens this latter concern, for all of a sudden the accepter is in the position of saying, in effect, "I know that this is likely to be a sensitive matter for you, but I must tell you that you have a serious problem that you may well have been ignorant about but that is serious enough that you must do something about it." Hence, in warning the other, the accepter is not only raising something that is apt to be the subject of insecurity but is also, in doing so, telling the other what to do. Accordingly, the warning—morally required though it is—seriously complicates the accepter's task of discharging his or her special responsibility for looking after the autonomy concerns connected with the privacy waiver. The question is, how can and should the accepter promote these autonomy concerns, once the warning has been given or once the sensitive issue has been broached?

Having taken on board the feminists' point that autonomy and agential self-confidence are never achieved by individuals in isolation but depend upon a nurturing background of familial and friendly relationships, we know that, in general, supporting these autonomy concerns is not always best carried out by backing off and allowing space for privacy. Sometimes it is best carried out by being a supportive interlocutor. These divergent means of supporting autonomy concerns are, in gross, mutually exclusive. It is hard to be supportive about matters from which one is backing off and leaving to the other to deal with alone, and conversely. The Charles Boyer character in "Gaslight" undercuts the agential self-confidence of Ingrid Bergman's not by prying but by being cruelly undercutting—the opposite of supportive. Confidence in one's ability to make up one's own mind, too, can be undercut by unsupportiveness.

Applying these observations now to the issue at hand, my claim is that the morally required warning (or broaching of the sensitive issue) has transformed this situation from one in which the best and most apt way of promoting these autonomy concerns would likely have been to back off and keep one's distance into one in which one is instead called upon to be supportive. The parties have unexpectedly come face-to-face with a vulnerability of the offeror's, one that requires some attention and one that the accepter can do something about. Especially if the offeror was unaware of his incompetence in cleaning the kitchen or of his gambling addiction, he will likely feel temporarily at a loss when suddenly confronted with the issue. It is particularly at such moments, when we are confronted with unexpected vulnerabilities, that we need some support in coming to our decisions. While we would typically prefer that such support come from our close intimates, broaching the issue *makes* the accepter an intimate of the offeror on this issue. Hence, the morally required warning (or broaching of the issue) likely converts the situation from one in which the accepter's heightened responsibility for the autonomy concerns calls for backing off to one in which it calls for tactful engagement. This is not to say that it calls for a helping response as such; still, the kind of engagement it does call for will still further deepen the relationship, further intensifying, rather than inhibiting, the special obligation of beneficence that attaches to it.

## How the Duty of Tactful Engagement Provides a Focus for Beneficence

As just noted, a special duty of tactful engagement is not equivalent to a special duty of care. Recall, however, that I have assumed, in the background, a specifiable duty of general beneficence. It is the conjunction of that duty with the duty of tactful engagement that supports a special ancillary-care duty in these cases of privacy-based moral entanglements. The special duty of tactfully engaging

with the offeror provides an apt circumstantial focus for specifying the general duty. Otherwise put, the general duty provides the
tilt towards active care that is needed to convert the special duty of
tactful engagement into a special ancillary-care duty.

Given this basis for special obligations of beneficence arising
out of intimacies, whether they actually require the accepter to offer
ancillary care will depend upon how the offeror wants to go about
addressing his or her need now that it has come out in the open. Once
having broached the issue, the accepter ought next to give the offeror
a chance either to ask for or to turn down one's help. If the offeror asks
for help, then the accepter should work with him or her in addressing the problem, where possible taking the lead from the offeror. The
accepter can avoid a paternalistic or condescending attitude by recognizing both that the other starts with certain definite ends in view
and that, since these are another's ends, one should generally defer to
the other's ways of revising and specifying them (cf. O'Neill, 1985,
271). The point is to work with the other on this delicate matter, letting
the other call the shots and thereby bolstering his or her threatened
autonomy by helping him or her exercise it. If the old man wants help
with the pile of mold, one should ask him how, specifically, one can
help him rather than simply grabbing a bottle of cleanser and tackling
the problem. In discussing medical researchers' ancillary-care obligations, people I think simply *assume* that the relevant care is wanted by
those who need it. While this may generally be a fair assumption, in
practice it will of course be important to check.

In sum, then, these privacy-based entanglements arise because
in accepting another's waiver of privacy rights, one takes on special
responsibility for the concerns underlying these rights. Once one has
warned the other about a new problem that one discovers on the basis
of private information (or has otherwise broached the issue), the morally best way to address these underlying concerns becomes not to
duck out, but rather to help the other address the problem—assuming

the other wants help. In this way, the duty to warn (or its cognates) further deepens the incipient relationship begun by the initial intimacy, providing a clear locus for a special obligation of beneficence. The upshot is a special ancillary-care obligation.

## RETURNING TO THE CONTEXT OF MEDICAL RESEARCH

The basis of the special ancillary-care obligation, then, lies in the special responsibility for protecting participants' autonomy that falls to researchers when they accept the participants' waivers of their privacy rights. In one respect, the argument applies even more strongly in the context of medical research than it does in many of the other cases of privacy-based moral entanglements that we have considered. In The Old Man and the Groceries, you are already helping the old man and the waiver of privacy was entirely at his initiative, yet this argument from the concerns underlying privacy still applies. This argument will apply all the more forcefully to cases in which the accepter has solicited a privacy waiver for his or her own purposes. One such case is The Reporter and the Peasant. Generally (albeit not as a necessary fact), medical research is like this: usually, the researchers solicit the privacy waivers by seeking informed consent from prospective participants.[21] Presumably, a case like Malaria Researchers and Schistosomiasis is like this: the malaria researchers would have recruited participants, seeking their informed consent. Since medical researchers generally need to solicit (and always need to obtain) privacy waivers from their research participants in order to proceed permissibly with their studies, this, too, is a potential case of a privacy-based moral

21. As Leif Wenar has pointed out to me, it is possible, and sometimes in fact happens, that individuals, and indeed entire communities, seek out participation in medical research.

entanglement. In such a case, the concerns I have identified apply especially starkly in that, once the study is up and running, these medical researchers have no professional reason to consider their participants as setters of ends. Instead, what they want from these people are just some biological samples or medical information. Against this backdrop, the privacy-based reasons to take account of potential threats to these people's autonomy shows up in more stark relief but also is all the more insistent, as the researchers must take care to treat the participants as autonomous persons and not as mere sources of biological materials.

Against this proposed account, it will reasonably be objected that not all ancillary medical needs that arise in medical research will pose a threat to the privacy waiver's confidence in his or her ability to set ends. The normal volunteer in Brain Scans who is unexpectedly told that he seems to have a brain tumor and needs urgent clinical follow-up to determine whether this is really so is apt to be quite bowled over by this discovery. By contrast, some diagnoses that researchers reach during the course of trials might not even bring any real news to the participants or might concern matters far less momentous than life-and-death.

I must recognize that there is some truth in this. I concede, for instance, that even if my participation in a study like that in the Brain Scan case ended up revealing a funny-looking and potentially worrisome blob in my brain, I would like to think that I would call my friends to identify the best neurologist to consult and would proceed to adjust my aims and plans according to what I found out. To this objection, though, I have four lines of response. First, confidence in one's ability to set ends is a matter of degree and always remains subject to setbacks. A second, more concessive point is that the test of strength put forward by the partial-entrustment model is available here to qualify or weaken a claim like mine. In responding in the way I hope I would, I would be indicating that I did not consider myself particularly dependent on these researchers for getting the care I need. Third, it is built into my account that ancillary care ought not to be pressed on an unwilling recipient. Hence, in cases where the person waiving the privacy rights is particularly secure against the given threat, merely offering a warning may suffice. Fourth, though, we should not want or expect moral principles to be fully tailored to all of the variations that can arise in individual cases. Just as the rationale for privacy rights is built on considerations that apply only by-and-large, so, too, the principles that apply to moral entanglements may be built on considerations that apply only by-and-large. This may mean that privacy-based entanglements arise fairly generally, even though the degree to which autonomy is threatened in any given case varies considerably.

My suggestion, then, is that what accounts for privacy-based moral entanglements in general, including those that arise in medical research, is that by voluntarily entering within the envelope, so to speak, of another's privacy protections, one becomes in a limited way liable to obligations to act to promote the fundamental interests those privacy protections normally protect. The discovery of an ancillary need can trigger a duty to warn and thereby activate these potential obligations, requiring one to cooperate with the other so as to address the need as—and if—the other would have one address it. In this way, the idea of privacy-based moral entanglements explains how participants in medical research entrust certain aspects of their health into the researchers' hands.

## POTENTIAL RIVAL ACCOUNTS: VULNERABILITY AND THREAT AVOIDANCE

My principal aim in the present chapter has been to put on the table an unrecognized and under-theorized type of moral consideration, one that explains how moral entanglements can arise from intimacies, defined as transactions that saliently involve the accepted waiver of privacy rights. My account gives these privacy waivers a central role in justifying the resulting moral entanglements. Some philosophers will find my account overly complex and will want to suggest that what is defensible in the intuitive phenomena of entanglement that I have laid out can be captured on the basis of simpler principles that avoid appealing to layers of directed claims and obligations. In accounting for moral phenomena, an undifferentiated consequentialism almost always offers the simplest possible approach, but not always an illuminating one. Here, I will instead very briefly consider two distinct rival accounts—each compatible at some level with consequentialism, but neither committed to it— one that focuses on the vulnerability of those who need help and one that focuses on who it is who can most easily neutralize threats. Each of these rival accounts of the phenomena of moral entanglement more generally—as laid out in the above cases—could also serve, more specifically, as a basis for an account of medical researchers' ancillary-care obligations.

According to a vulnerability theory of helping obligations, help should go to the most vulnerable. Following Robert Goodin, the premier defender of such a theory, we can think of vulnerability, here, in a relatively rigorous way as "being under threat of harm" (Goodin, 1985, 110). By threatened harm, Goodin does not mean harm that someone has threatened in an attempt to get someone to do something, but more generally harm that would be averted if someone or other acts in a certain way. The potential victim's well-being is thus in some way at stake and is—as he puts it—"vulnerable to" what one or more other people choose to do (33, 163n.). Rather than seeking simply to add a distinct sort of moral consideration alongside rescue and promissory obligations, as I have done here, Goodin sought to demonstrate that the obligation to respond to vulnerability underlies all of our special obligations (33). His intuitive entrée into this project was the obligations of parents to their children. "The most salient feature of the human infant," he remarks, "is its severe and protracted vulnerability." Of course, someone in particular must be assigned the responsibility to care for children. Lots of different adults could remove the threats to any given child; but "[w]ho that is will, of course, be a matter for social determination" (33). Vulnerability gives rise to the fundamental moral pull; the further social details are secondary.

A focus on vulnerability will take one a considerable way through my cases of intimacies, including all of the cases of ancillary-care needs that I have mentioned in previous chapters. In all of the cases I have raised, I have spoken of ancillary-care needs that the other party in the intimacy can effectively address. Hence, in every one of my cases, the person with the ancillary-care need is "vulnerable to" the other in Goodin's specific sense, which is also the sense adopted by the partial-entrustment model's test of strength. Furthermore, given the existence of the intimacy, it generally makes sense, at some social level, to assign responsibility for addressing needy persons' absolute vulnerabilities to others with whom they are in this way intimate.

To confine the explanation only to my cases of intimacies in this way, however, is to miss an important distinction implicit in them. Except in the two variants of the Massage Therapist case, I have not taken space to spell out contrasting cases. Throughout, however, my argument in this chapter has been that intimacies give rise to *heightened* duties of care—heightened, that is, compared to the general, non-transactional baseline. For each of my other cases, I would claim, there are counterpart cases in which the vulnerabilities are identical and the ancillary-care duties absent because no intimacy has been created. Like the massage therapist in the dropped-towel variant of that case, a tax accountant who happened to see a pattern indicative of gambling addiction in a stranger's and non-client's financial records that mistakenly came his way will not, I claim, have special ancillary-care obligations to this stranger. Similarly with a medical researcher who happened to see schisto-somiasis parasites in a microscope image carelessly left around by another research group. My arguments in the previous section have explained the moral difference between the cases. The vulnerability theory, straightforwardly interpreted, tends to imply that there should not be such a moral difference between these cases. Hence, I claim, it does not fully fit the relevant phenomena.

Possibly, however, the defender of the vulnerability theory would want to try to capture this complexity of the appearances.[22] In doing so, the vulnerability theory's flexible views about to whom, in particular, responsibilities should be assigned can be put to work. There are social costs involved in letting strange accountants or strange doctors poke through one's private information, and hence social reasons to inhibit acting on information one has obtained without permission, even if blamelessly. These social costs could be invoked in order to fit, to a large extent, the more complex pattern of appearances that I allege.

I do not doubt this possibility, but I suspect that to make it work, the social costs involved will have to be quite heavily moralized ones. They will need to include the dangers of strange accountants and doctors and grocery-bag carriers sticking their noses into what is really not their business. That is, they will include the dangers

---

22. There is another way the vulnerability theorist might set out to capture some of the appearances, one that has been suggested to me by some comments of Robert Goodin's. Perhaps one has an obligation to help everyone one can whenever one can—everyone who is relationally vulnerable to you—so long as one can do so without violating their rights. In some cases, this will mean that unless a person has waived some privacy rights, one has no obligation to help him or her. While this route does look like it might well explain most of the appearances, I find implausible its presupposition of an unlimited obligation of permissible aid.

of intrusions on privacy rights. If this is the way things go, I am inclined to say: I recognize the force of the idea of vulnerability, but would like to do more to unpack the moral considerations here being lumped together under the rubric of social cost. That is part of what my account aims to do.

As appealing as the call to address vulnerability is, it is one-sided in its victim- or patient-centeredness. Leif Wenar's least-cost threat avoider (LCTA) view, by contrast, is more agent-centered because it offers an individualistic, as opposed to social, account of whose obligation it is to address a given threat (Wenar, 2007; cf. Miller, 2001). Whereas the message of the vulnerability view is that people's vulnerabilities must be attended to in a socially efficacious way, the message of the LCTA view is that if there is a threat that ought to be averted and if you are the person who can most easily avert it, then—modulo certain provisos—you have an obligation to do so. Barbara Herman (2001, 231) has gone so far as to assert that "[n]ormally, in providing aid, we take on new responsibilities." The LCTA view can explain why this would be so on an appealingly simple, pragmatic basis. By starting to help people, one learns a considerable amount about them and their plight. This increment in knowledge, combined with a continued proximity, may imply that one is a person who can deal particularly (or most) easily with yet other aspects of their plight. As Wenar has developed this view, it is addressed principally to the question of how to "locate responsibility for any particular task" (2007, 256). Having in mind a task whose urgency is relatively self-evident—that of alleviating severe poverty—Wenar develops what he calls "the least-cost principle" to address the question of which agents are responsible for urgent tasks of averting threats (2007, 265; cf. 261).

Wenar does not intend us to take the "least cost" language too literally. He initially states his principle as holding that "the agent who most easily can avert the threat [to an individual's 'basic well-being'] has the responsibility for doing so" (2007, 260). Again, because the view takes the urgency of a given threat for granted, it is not intended to guide individuals who are forced to choose which of two threats to avert—a fairly serious threat that they can easily avert or a more serious threat that they can avert with somewhat more trouble. Sticking with a given threat, however, I do take it that the view is meant to take account of variables such as the completeness with which an agent is able to avert a threat and the probability that an agent will succeed in averting a threat to a given extent.

Understanding the view this way, we can see that it can cope with the facts of my main cases even more flexibly than can the vulnerability view. The principal reason for this is that the LCTA view is more directly sensitive to the potential helper's epistemic position. The intimacies of most of my examples have put the potential helpers in a distinctive position of knowing about the other's predicament. That already contributes a lot to the ease with which they could help. The young man who has carried in the bags in the case of The Old Man and the Groceries, for instance, is in a presumptively unique position of knowing about the threat posed by the festering mold. Getting someone else in there to deal with it is likely to be a lot less easy than his taking care of it himself.

Now, before I state my principal response to the LCTA view, I would like to repeat a point that I made in response to the vulnerability view. Given that we are interpreting the LCTA view rather loosely, there will be some temptation to read it in a way that takes account of moral costs. The young man has already been invited into the old man's home, and so can make observations about the state of the old man's countertops without being a complete buttinsky. Others who set out to avoid this kind of threat would have to cook up pretexts to enter the apartments of the elderly, going to some costly efforts to arrange to discover hygiene problems. This contrast is part of what makes it relatively easy for the young man of my initial example to intervene. To this, my response is that this is of course so, and is explained by the prior privacy waiver. As I said about the vulnerability view so interpreted: If the LCTA view is developed this way, I may not disagree with it. What I would want to do, though, is to linger longer over the unpacking of these moral costs, which are shifted by the unfolding moral transactions between the parties. That, again, is what my account has tried to do.

My principal response to the LCTA view, however, has to do not with explaining which of several potential threat averters ought to avert a threat but with whether anyone has an obligation to avert a given threat. Like the general duty of rescue, the LCTA's general duty will have a threshold of costliness. If there is no potential threat averter for whom the cost falls below the threshold, then no one will have a duty to avert the threat. In keeping with the general spirit of the LCTA view, we might suppose that this threshold would be impartially set. But the moral difference that a waiver of privacy rights makes can help explain not only why one person rather than another should be the designated threat averter: It can also help explain why in one situation there exists someone with a duty to avert the threat and in another situation there does not. That is, this aspect of the transactional history between two individuals can explain why, in a non-impartial or transaction-sensitive way, the threshold should be set differently in one case than in another.

Speaking in this way about which important threats must morally be met assumes that not all of them must be. Unfortunately, this is the case. In some tragic cases that arise in medical research, for instance, the ancillary-care need that arises is one that would be prohibitively expensive for anyone to address. One such case, Advanced Cervical Cancer in a HIV-transmission Study, was mentioned in Chapter 1. In that case, researchers in a longitudinal observational study of HIV-AIDS transmission in western Uganda who were looking specifically at the effect of sexually transmitted diseases on HIV-transmission rates found advanced cervical cancer in one of the participants while doing a physical exam for STDs. Unfortunately, there was no surgeon in Uganda capable of doing the surgery she needed to save her life. Dickert and Wendler (2009) report that the echocardiograms conducted on participants in Mali during the study of malaria and pulmonary hypertension on which they focused discovered a life-threatening heart defect (a ventricular septal defect) in one of the participating children. Again, unfortunately, there was no cardiothoracic surgeon in Mali to whom they could refer the child. At the time of their writing, these authors report, the researchers were still trying to see if they could arrange for donors to fly the child to Europe for surgery. As these cases dramatize, we cannot simply assume that all urgent medical needs will, or even "must," be met. As I have said, I am here steering clear of the kind of ideal theory that would first insist that the world's allocation of resources be just.

The vulnerability view and the LCTA view are one-sided, then, in opposite ways, the former focusing on the victims and the latter focusing on the potential helpers. While each captures a type of consideration important to our overall set of helping obligations, they leave out crucially relevant facts that arise from transactions between pairs of people, a potential helper and a potential victim. Clearly, a transactional view like mine needs to be sensitive both to relative levels of vulnerability and to the relative ease or cost of helping. Although absolute levels of cost or of the other's resources can limit intimacy-based ancillary-care obligations, the transactional considerations that underlie these obligations can clearly support a shift in one's helping priorities, away from what an approach that is impartial about vulnerabilities and costs would dictate. For example, in Malaria Researchers and Schistosomiasis, it may well be that the individuals who have managed to get themselves enrolled in such a malaria study are relatively well off, compared to the truly destitute and also malaria- and schistosomiasis-ridden people who live too far from town centers to have been able to participate in a malaria trial. This kind of possibility raises issues of justice that have been discussed by Merritt and Grady (2006) and that I will take up in the following chapter. Although the researchers might theoretically steer their help towards these non-participants, their more demanding intimacy-based obligation gives the researchers a significant moral reason to give priority to their study participants.

On the account defended in this chapter, significant intimacy-based moral entanglements flow from a distinctive sort of moral transaction. In contrast to promising, whereby we can voluntarily extend our obligations in ways that are largely under the control of our own wills, voluntarily entering into intimacies by accepting privacy waivers can extend our obligations in ways that we do not intend or foresee. What explains why this is so, I have argued, is that one takes on some responsibility for addressing the moral considerations underlying privacy rights when one has accepted another's waiver of privacy rights and that these responsibilities morph when one has warned the other about a danger discovered on the basis of private information. To enter into a potentially entangling intimacy of this kind, one must voluntarily exercise this moral power. This makes the resulting obligations special in the sense I defined at the outset: dependent on the history of transactions between the people in question. We have seen that such privacy-based moral entanglements arise in a wide variety of contexts, professional and casual. In medical research, as I argued in the previous chapter, the acceptance of the participants' privacy waivers defines the outset of the researcher–participant relationship. The present chapter's argument explains why these privacy waivers matter, morally, setting out how the acceptance of privacy waivers gives rise to special obligations of ancillary care.

# Chapter 4

# Justice, Exploitation, and Ancillary Care

I have said that, in developing my account of medical researchers' special ancillary-care obligations, I would not be imagining away the significant background injustices that hinder the access of many around the world to adequate health care. These injustices include the effects of past conquest, colonization, exploitation, and looting; the ongoing effects of skewed principles of international commercial law (e.g., Pogge, 2007); and ongoing cases of theft or inadequately authorized appropriation of the natural resources rightly belonging to the oppressed peoples of the world (Wenar, 2008). In addition, woefully inadequate access to health care arguably counts as a human rights violation, and hence as an injustice, unto itself.[1] Because idealizing away such injustices would—I argued—amount to shutting one's eyes to many of the most urgent existing needs for ancillary care, idealizing in this way would be a mistake in developing an account of our moral responsibilities in the context of these needs.

Especially with such injustices in the background, to say that medical researchers and their sponsors have important ancillary-care obligations that they specially owe to their research participants is *not* to say that we, the citizens of the world—and especially

1. See, e.g., U.N. General Assembly (2008). For broad, philosophical treatments of justice in health care, see, e.g., Powers & Faden (2006), Daniels (2007), and Ruger (2010).

we, the educated and relatively affluent citizens of the world—are off the hook with regard to everyone else who is needy. Of course we have a duty to help rectify these injustices and ameliorate the conditions of abject poverty and deep oppression to which they have given rise! As I have repeatedly done in this book, I am here again suggesting that we see medical researchers' special ancillary-care obligations as supplementing any general obligations that they and others have. These include any obligations of justice they have—wherever they live—as relatively affluent and privileged citizens of the world.

I recognize, then, the deep problems of background justice that especially afflict those in developing countries, both because of global injustice and as a domestic legacy of colonial and other forms of oppression. I insist that duties arising with regard to these injustices—such as those relevant for medical researchers captured by the pragmatic priority for "relief of oppression" urged by Lavery et al. (2010)—could coherently supplement any special ancillary-care obligation. This stance, however, will not satisfy everyone. Some will want to see an account of ancillary-care obligations grounded more directly in considerations of justice. For instance, Solomon Benatar and Peter A. Singer, in a reprise discussion of these issues of justice in international medical research, which they had first raised in a classic article of ten years before (Benatar & Singer, 2000), find fault with my approach on these grounds. They bring it up together with the "fair benefits" approach, which generally concerns post-trial benefits, such as making a successful trial drug available on an ongoing basis (Emanuel et al., 2004). Benatar and Singer suggest that "[w]hile these approaches are of value, they have been criticized as being focused on micro-conceptions of exploitation and thus limited to a thin conception of justice (procedural in nature) to be applied on a case-by-case basis and without taking account of background conditions of injustice."[2] It is true that I suggest that we look at the special ancillary-care obligation in a way that is focused—in a "micro" fashion—on the transactions between particular researchers (or research teams) and individual research participants; and it is also true that I suggest that this issue be treated separately from the underlying issues of background injustice. It is important to consider whether this is a mistake. Perhaps considerations of justice ought to be integrated more fully into our understanding of researchers' special ancillary-care obligations.

Questions of justice might—and do—impinge on ancillary-care issues in many different ways. We must distinguish between whether considerations of justice can *ground* medical researchers' special ancillary-care obligations and whether considerations of justice *shape or constrain* those obligations in important ways. In the first, negative part of this chapter, I will argue that considerations of justice cannot serve to ground these special obligations. In doing so, I will explain why Benatar and Singer are mistaken in expecting the partial-entrustment model of this special obligation to handle the issue of exploitation. In the second section, I will discuss three different ways in which acting on the special ancillary-care obligation can itself raise worries about injustice. One of these, the apparent injustice of "burdening the helper," was already addressed in the previous chapter. The other two are the important worries about "undue inducement" of study participation and the challenging issues that arise in relation to giving study participants priority over other needy people. Finally, in the third section, I will discuss

2. Benatar & Singer (2010), p. 194, citing Ballantyne (2008), whose critique is actually directed only against the "fair benefits approach." Benatar and Singer, however, apparently take it also to apply to the approach to ancillary care that I developed with Belsky. They immediately go on to suggest how one might "rectify" this "shortcoming."

in a more general way how duties of justice can reinforce ancillary-care obligations.

## WHY SPECIAL ANCILLARY-CARE OBLIGATIONS CANNOT REST ON JUSTICE

The reason why medical researchers' special ancillary-care obligations cannot rest on justice is quite abstract and is reasonably simple. The relevant duties of justice—duties of distributive justice—are not special duties, but instead are owed to anyone in specified circumstances, irrespective of the transactional history between the two people. There are special duties of justice; but these are duties of rectificatory justice, which are not generally relevant in the context of ancillary care.[3] As I explained in Chapter 1, my central aim in this book is to explain the nature and grounds of the special ancillary-care obligation that medical researchers owe to the participants in their studies. General duties of distributive justice have the wrong structure to ground such a special duty, while special duties of rectificatory justice have the wrong content.[4] Let me spell out each of these points in turn.

"Principles of distributive justice," according to one standard definition, "are normative principles designed to guide the allocation of the benefits and burdens of economic activity" (Lamont & Favor, 2007). Principles may do so either directly, by indicating what should be allocated to whom, or indirectly, by constraining basic social and economic institutions that determine the allocation

---

3. Not *generally* relevant: for an illustration of the reason for this qualification, see the case of Quinodyne, below.
4. I rest my argument on these two familiar notions, distributive justice and rectificatory justice. I do not purport to say what justice, as such, involves. In taking such a stance, I am imitating Aristotle: see his *Nicomachean Ethics*, Book V, Chapters 2–4.

of economic benefits and burdens. Thus, for example, John Rawls (2001, 50) insists on distinguishing his institutional account of distributive justice from more narrowly "allocative" accounts. In considering whether principles of distributive justice might help generate or ground medical researchers' special ancillary-care obligations, it makes sense to concentrate on more narrowly "allocative" principles, since these at least directly concern what individuals should get. Hence, we should put aside an institutional principle such as the following:

> *Institutional basic minimum:* All individuals should strive to see to it that every society (or: their own societies) guarantees to all of its citizens a minimally decent standard of living (including a decent minimum of access to health care).

Instead, we should focus our attention on more narrowly allocative principles, such as this one:

> *Allocative basic minimum:* All individuals should strive to see to it that everyone has access to a minimally decent standard of living (including a decent minimum of access to health care).

This principle, like the foregoing, is simple and stark, and might or might not need considerable qualification to be plausible as a principle of justice.[5] In interpreting this latter principle for practical purposes, one would naturally note that some people are in a better

5. Rawls, I take it, would support principles at least roughly similar to these, in light of (a) his support for a principle requiring that social institutions meet "citizens' basic needs...at least insofar as their being met is necessary for citizens to understand and to be able fruitfully to exercise [their basic] rights and liberties" (Rawls, 1996, p. 7) and (b) his support for a "natural duty of justice" applicable to individuals, which holds, in part, that "we are to assist in the establishment of just arrangements where they do not exist" (Rawls, 1999b, pp. 293–294).

position than others to make efforts in this direction. In particular, we relatively wealthy and educated individuals can do more to lobby for reforms in this direction and to donate to organizations devoted to this kind of effort than can others. Even so, this principle applies to *all* individuals, and does not pick out any of them specially, whether on the basis of some past transaction with the deprived or otherwise. As such, it is not the kind of principle that would be able to explain why medical researchers, *as researchers* (and not simply as relatively educated and affluent people), have a special duty to their research participants, *as their research participants*, and not simply as poor and deprived people whose basic needs are not met.

It may be objected that one familiar type of theory of distributive justice, namely Robert Nozick's libertarian theory, illustrates that principles of distributive justice can focus on the transactional histories between individuals. Here is Nozick's ideal theory of "justice in holdings" (1974, 151):

1. A person who acquires a holding in accordance with the principle of justice in acquisition is entitled to that holding.
2. A person who acquires a holding in accordance with the principle of justice in transfer, from someone else entitled to the holding, is entitled to the holding.
3. No one is entitled to a holding except by (repeated) applications of 1 and 2.

Now, it is certainly true that Nozick's account of distributive justice is "historical" or transactional at the core. Notice, however, that it does not state or directly imply any duties of any kind. Rather, it articulates rights. Duties enter Nozick's picture in the way indicated by his book's famous opening lines: "Individuals have rights, and there are things no person or group may do to them (without violating their rights). So strong and far-reaching are these rights that they raise the question of what, if anything, the state and its officials may do" (1974, ix). The duty not to violate anyone's entitlements in holding is, again, a perfectly general obligation incumbent on everyone, independently of one's transactional history with this or that particular person. Conversely, if an individual's claim to hold a given piece of property is invalid because he acquired it by force, this fact tends to imply that *no one* has a duty to respect his ownership thereof. In this regard, the person from whom the property was forcibly wrested (even if still alive) is not in a morally different position from anyone else. What this shows is that even Nozick's ideal transactional theory of distributive justice is not transactional in the right way to give rise to special duties.

Of course, as Nozick forthrightly admitted, his ideal transactional theory is manifestly incomplete, since so much of the past history of the world is riddled with injustice in original acquisition and injustice in the transfer of holdings. Given the historical nature of his transactional theory, he thus was obliged to include within his account of distributive justice a principle of "rectification of injustice in holdings." This principle, which he did not specify, would address such questions as the following (Nozick, 1974, 152):

> If past injustice has shaped present holdings in various ways, some identifiable and some not, what now, if anything, ought to be done to rectify these injustices? What obligations do the performers of injustice have toward those whose position is worse than it would have been if the injustice had not been done?

While Nozick thus ranged this principle of rectification under the heading of distributive justice, it is clear that questions of rectificatory justice can also arise independently, such as when one's concern is simply with theft and duress, and not with the society-wide set of holdings.[6] A principle of rectificatory justice that arises within an account of distributive justice will either indicate what "the performers of injustice" owe to those they have made worse off or it will not. If it does not, then it will represent some form of adjustment to the ideal transactional theory. For instance, it might take the form of an exception or proviso appended to clause (3), to yield something like the following:

3*. No one is entitled to a holding except by (repeated) applications of 1 and 2, except that where there has been a pervasive history of unjust acquisition and unjust transfer that has benefited the wealthy (or, the capitalists, or the colonizers, or...), the poor (or, the workers, or the colonized, or...) are entitled to redistributional support from the state, financed by progressive taxation.

Here, I am not interested in the merits of such a principle, but only in its form. The point is, this is still a fully general principle of distributive justice, giving rise only to general duties. If, by contrast, the principle of rectification Nozick called for instead—or also—addressed what obligations individual transgressors owe to those against whom they have transgressed, then that would put this rectificatory component of his distributive theory on the same footing as ordinary principles of rectificatory justice. Accordingly, I turn now to those.

Medical researchers can certainly owe duties of rectificatory justice to their study participants. For instance, they will arguably owe them such duties whenever they have negligently harmed the participants. In the context of medical research, failures and

---

6. This, of course, is Aristotle's way of introducing the topic of rectificatory justice at the outset of *Nicomachean Ethics* V.4.

irregularities in the informed-consent process count as, or provide evidence for, criticizable negligence on the part of the researchers. Such failures of process were found by the FDA to have occurred in the gene-therapy trials in which Jesse Gelsinger died in 1999.[7] Where researcher negligence of this kind or any other has led to research participants being injured as a result of participating in a trial, the researchers owe these participants compensation as a matter of rectificatory (a.k.a. compensatory) justice. Claims to such compensation are morally very weighty and no doubt would take precedence, where the two clash, over many ancillary-care claims. Here, my narrow point about these claims to compensation, however, is that they cannot directly ground claims to ancillary care. That is because, as I have defined ancillary care, it is "medical care that the research subjects need but that is not required to make a study scientifically valid, to ensure a study's safety, or to redress research injuries." This definition thus puts into a different category all claims to compensation for injury, whether grounded in negligence, intentional harming, or non-criticizable accident. Care that a participant needs as a result of a trial-caused injury or illness is, by definition, not ancillary care. Putting duties of compensation in a different category than ancillary-care duties make sense, as the former derive from violations of principles of non-maleficence or justice and the latter are more plausibly seen as belonging to the family of beneficence principles.

There is another way that duties of rectificatory justice might be relevant to medical researchers' ancillary-care obligations. Some of those obligations could derive from injustices committed against groups, rather than against individuals. Such a possibility has been

---

7. See the letter of Feb. 8, 2002, from Dennis E. Baker, Associate Commissioner of the FDA for Regulatory Affairs, to Dr. James M. Wilson, available at http://www.fda.gov/downloads/RegulatoryInformation/FOI/ElectronicReadingRoom/UCM144544.pdf (accessed July 18, 2010).

explored by Hooper (2010). Building on his observations, let me given an example, guided by the thought that principles of rectificatory justice might apply to researchers as individuals from—or sponsored by—a colonizing nation who are doing research in a former colony. They might apply to them as individuals who have indirectly benefited from their country's past unfair exploitation of the resource riches of the country in which they are now conducting their research. Let us imagine such a case, involving a hypothetical pharmaceutical company, Quinodyne. Based in the Netherlands, this imaginary multinational giant had its beginnings in the early 20th-century exploitation of quinine in the Indonesian archipelago. While Quinodyne was perhaps no worse than other colonial exploiters of its day, its treatment of the workers on its quinine plantations was abusive and its impact on the local economy was ultimately—let us suppose—quite ruinous. Now, though, Quinodyne is back in Java, this time running a trial of its new asthma drug. This population of research subjects is no longer among the very poorest of the world. Arguments of distributive justice thus do not apply as strongly here as they would in some other places. What may get a better grip, in this case, are arguments of rectificatory justice. Quinodyne arguably owes some reparations to the descendants of its Javanese quinine laborers. Since it is now back in Indonesia as a sponsor of drug research, it would not be inappropriate for those reparations to take the form of extended post-trial drug availability or, as it may be, superlative ancillary care.

I will return to duties of rectificatory justice in the final section of this chapter, in order to look at how such duties may reinforce researchers' special ancillary-care responsibilities. For now, though, I stick with the question whether such duties can ground special ancillary-care obligations. Again, my answer is no. Although such duties might ground obligations that these researchers owe to these research participants, these are not duties that apply to the researchers *as researchers*. "Ancillary care" is defined relative to research (or, in the more abstract fashion of Chapter 3, relative to the point of the privacy-waiving interaction between the parties). What counts as ancillary care from the point of view of a medical researcher will simply count as ordinary clinical care from the point of view of a person's primary-care physician. Insofar as we are talking about obligations to provide ancillary medical care, then, we are talking about obligations that medical researchers have *as researchers*. Hence, while they might be special duties in the sense that they derive from the particular history of the sponsoring nation and the host nation, they are not specially focused on the researchers and participants. And it has been, all along, an obligation that researchers specially owe to their participants that I have been mainly attempting to analyze.

In short, duties of distributive justice are too general to serve as the basis of medical researchers' ancillary-care obligations, while duties of rectificatory justice, though special, are either irrelevant to ancillary care by definition or else are not specifically focused on researchers and research participants as such.

Since ancillary-care issues thus involve considerations quite different from issues of justice, it would also be a mistake to try to use an ancillary-care theory like the partial-entrustment account as a basis for trying to address issues of justice. The partial-entrustment model of researchers' ancillary-care responsibilities is not intended to help us deal generally with the issues of justice and exploitation that arise within the context of medical research. The partial-entrustment model picks up on *a* central feature of the researcher–participant relationship without making any claim that it is, for all purposes, the most central feature thereof. It seems to me no defect of the partial-entrustment model that it does not generate an account of exploitation, just as it is no defect of a fork that it is ill suited to drinking soup. In being designed to generate an account of unjust exploitation, the "fair benefits" approach differs in aim from the partial-entrustment model. For this reason, it was odd of Benatar and Singer to lump the two together as approaches to exploitation—ones that (allegedly) stick too much with "micro" issues.

That the partial-entrustment model does not provide a basis for accounting for unjust exploitation is thus not a defect of the account. What *would* be a defect of the account, however, would be if following it would generate more exploitation or injustice than otherwise exists. I turn to this sort of worry next.

## WILL PROVIDING ANCILLARY CARE CONFLICT WITH JUSTICE?

One worry about exploitation that the partial-entrustment model raises—albeit not one in the spirit of the other concerns about justice raised so far in this chapter—is that its specification of researchers' ancillary-care obligations will end up dictating that the *researchers* be exploited. This worry is the one raised by the "burdening the helper" objection addressed in the previous chapter. Researchers might complain that it was unjust that, on top of all of their efforts and personal sacrifice in the cause of finding a malaria vaccine or a way to slow HIV transmission in Africa or...they were also being asked to provide or arrange ancillary care for their participants. The previous chapter developed an answer to this objection at such length that the reader may have missed it, so I will sum it up here. As that chapter's broader discussion of privacy-based moral entanglements indicated, that is just the way it goes when one voluntarily accepts someone's waivers of privacy rights: one lets oneself in for additional, special responsibilities whose practical demands one cannot fully predict.

More in tune with the concerns about justice raised so far in this chapter is the worry that instituting ancillary-care obligations would exacerbate existing exploitation of poor and vulnerable research participants by providing them additional inducements to participate. There is considerable concern about "undue inducement" of study participation, especially where the pool of participants is uneducated or desperately poor. That concern can arise simply from the fact that the study offers study-related clinical care or from its offering cash incentives "or some item of value such as a shirt, toothbrush, or transport of a casket for burial" for participation (Emanuel, Currie, & Herman, 2005, 337). Adding ancillary care to the package of benefits that a potential participant can expect intensifies this concern.

At a conceptual level, the careful distinctions developed by Ezekiel Emanuel and colleagues build a convincing case that undue inducement is never a serious moral concern just on its own (Emanuel, 2004; Emanuel, Currie, & Herman, 2005). It is only when extremely attractive offers are made in the context of some other injustice or some other important violation of medical research ethics that these offers become "undue inducement." Absent some such independent moral problem in the background, it is difficult to see what is morally problematic about an especially attractive offer. An offer does not become coercive or autonomy-undercutting just because it is one that the person who receives it will almost surely choose to accept. One type of independent moral problem, which can arguably explain why some offers give rise to undue inducement, is presumably *not* relevant in the context of medical research. This is the kind of problem that arises because the offer attempts to overcome the offeree's moral scruples. Extremely attractive offers can induce corruption. In the case of political bribery, we have rules against this, and for good reason, as we seek more generally to keep what Rawls called "the curse of money" (1999a, 139) at a distance from democratic decision-making. Political corruption, and more generally the kind of unequal influence on the political process that comes from throwing money around with contributions legal and illegal, does not merely undermine our faith in the political process. It also seems to bother us intrinsically.

We might similarly worry about corrupting offers in the context of medical research. Thus, imagine the following case:

> *A Transfusion for a Jehovah's Witness:* Suppose that researcher R is attempting to recruit A to be a participant in an interventional trial involving a rare disease from which A is suffering. The intervention, however, requires the participants to receive blood transfusions, and A indicates that, as a Jehovah's Witness, he has religious objections to receiving transfusions. Because, however, this particular disease is relatively common among Jehovah's Witnesses, R is prepared with a response. "We will pay you $5,000 if, despite these religious objections, you participate in this trial, including undergoing the transfusions it requires."

It might well be debated whether there is a moral problem with this offer (cf. Wertheimer, 2003, 171–177). If there is, it would be because it attempts to induce A to violate a moral principle (or something A considers to be one). But this is surely not a kind of worry that is particularly relevant in the medical-research contexts in which the issue of undue inducement comes up. The case just given is quite unrealistic. It is possible that specific cultures might have a more general moral ban on participating in medical research, such that individual members of those cultures had moral scruples about such participation that heavy inducements might overcome. Given the emphasis of the medical-research establishment on informed consent, however, it seems likely that researchers would steer away from working in such cultures. In any case, for the most part, when people raise worries about undue inducement to partici-pate in research, they are not usually worried about participants' moral scruples being overcome.

What worries people, under the heading of undue induce-ment to participate in research, is that poor and vulnerable people will get sucked into research that imposes undue risks on them. Powerful sponsors of research, whether corporations, govern-ments, or NGOs, are capable of throwing around their economic power in developing-country or inner-city settings, overwhelming potential participants' perhaps justified doubts about the wisdom of participating in a trial by sweetening the pot with cash or with offers of medical care, whether trial-related or ancillary. When one combines the fact that these research sponsors have vastly more access to financial resources than these potential participants with the equally relevant fact that these sponsors have vastly more access to information about the risks of the study procedures, one gets a fuller picture of the situation's dangers.

At the outset of this chapter, I noted that we live surrounded by pervasive background injustices. It is no stretch of the imagination to see the asymmetries of financial power and informational access I have just noted as generally manifesting these injustices. Had the history of the world not been shot through with unjust conquest, looting, and theft and were the international economic regime under which we live fully fair, such dramatic asymmetries might well not exist. Hence, even if one concedes to Emanuel and colleagues that extremely attractive offers of research participation pose no moral problem *in themselves*, there is never a shortage of background prob-lems of injustice with which such offers might combine in order to yield a morally worrisome situation. At a conceptual level, then, concerns about undue inducement cannot be written off even if, absent some independent moral problem, extremely attractive offers are never in themselves morally problematic.

Suppose this analysis is right at the conceptual level. The question then is, at a more practical level, how to address the remaining worries about undue inducement to participate in research. Presumably, the answer to this question should depend on why it is that the induced choices are likely to be regrettable ones. I have suggested that the answer to this is likely not that the participants' moral scruples have been overcome, in the fashion of A Transfusion for a Jehovah's Witness. Rather, what tends to be worrisome about many of the participants' choices is that they may have unwisely let themselves in for a level of risk that they have not adequately understood. At this practical level, then, the undue-inducement worry seems to call for a balanced, two-pronged response. The first prong is procedural. As Emanuel and colleagues emphasize, IRB and REC review of proposed trials should see to it that no medical study poses undue risks to participants. If this review is not succeeding in this goal, it may need to be tightened up in some way. Relatedly, these entities should also see to it that the informed-consent process adequately informs prospective participants of the risks that there are. If this goal could be achieved, the worry about undue inducement to participate in medical research would, I expect, largely fade away. Yet these ideals have been out there for some time, and abuses and lapses continue to occur in medical research: Undue risks continue to be imposed and informed consent can still be imperfect. Hence, this procedural approach needs to be supplemented by some substantive limits. This is the second prong. IRBs and RECs need to take a sensible, context-sensitive, and community-informed approach to what counts as a worrisome inducement. If researchers offered cash payments equivalent to several years' worth of an individual's otherwise expected income, that would raise a red flag. So, too, would committing in advance to fly participants to neighboring countries for any surgery necessary to address any ancillary-care need.

While I thus concede that, in the context of the great background injustices with which our world is afflicted, ancillary care can sometimes count as an undue inducement to participate in research, I would also argue that generally it does not. Compare the issue of an adequate "standard of care" for the disease or condition under study. People have gotten used to the idea that a reasonable standard of care for study participants is a core part of what is required in order to do research ethically. For that reason, there seems to be little tendency to take care offered in order to provide a reasonable standard of care for the disease or condition under study as providing undue inducement to trial participation. Nor should people worry about this: Generally speaking, the higher the level of care, the lower the risks of trial participation. The case is nearly parallel with ancillary care. The moral argument for ancillary care is on a par with that for a decent standard of care. Provision of ancillary care, too, should be regarded as a core requirement of doing medical research ethically. Now, it is true that ancillary care will not lower "study risks" the way that a good "standard of care" for the target disease or condition will; but ancillary care will lower the risk that participants will have unfortunate health outcomes. Hence, as a practical matter, I conclude that IRBs and RECs—as well as regulatory bodies and governmental watchdogs—should deal with the undue-inducement worries raised by offers of ancillary care not only in the substantive but context-sensitive way of the second prong, above, but also by emphasizing the first, procedural prong. That is to say, they should do what they can to see to it that studies involving undue risks to participants are not approved and are not conducted. To the extent that this aim can be secured, worries about undue inducement can be put to the side, and priority can be given to providing participants the care they ought to receive.

A final way in which provision of ancillary care threatens to interfere with justice raises the question, from a different angle, as to whether trial participants really do have a claim to receiving special care. Everywhere, resources available for medical care are scarce in relation to the potential needs. Everywhere, but especially in poor and poorly insured communities around the world, systems are in place to establish reasonably impartial ways of giving priority to those who most urgently need care. In a capitalist developed country such as the United States, these systems have to cope with the ways that the sheer purchasing power of a few can disrupt the ideal of allocating medical care in accordance with need. Even so, in hospital emergency rooms, for instance, the ideal of impartial allocation of medical resources to those who most urgently need them lives on. In many of the poorest developing nations, the principal threats to impartial allocation are different, and derive instead from arbitrary breakdowns in infrastructure, from political cronyism that ends up favoring those in some districts over others, and from the agendas of well-meaning foreigners who supply aid targeted to some diseases and not to others. Despite such challenges, many such nations have striven to implement fair ways of allocating such scarce medical commodities as antiretroviral treatments (ART) for treating HIV-AIDS. Merritt and Grady (2006, 1791) note that the legitimacy of each nation thus coming up with its own priorities in allocating ARTs is widely recognized. These national priorities, if fairly crafted and within reasonable bounds, establish what would count, in that country, as a just allocation of ARTs.[8] Let me illustrate this with an example. Suppose that a given developing nation's scheme for allocating ARTs gives priority—as the World Health Organization (WHO) has said it should—to "the most vulnerable,

---

8. On the idea that justice admits of local specification, see Aquinas (1981, Vol. II, 1914: I-II, Q. 95, Art. 2), Nussbaum (2000, 77), and Richardson (2008b).

poor and marginalized populations and for women" (WHO, 2004). And suppose that foreign-sponsored HIV researchers have, for sound scientific reasons, chosen to conduct a study of the effect of male circumcision on HIV transmission that will enroll males living in the capital. An ancillary-care argument for prioritizing these study participants over others—which, as I will indicate in Chapter 6, is likely to be quite compelling—threatens to disrupt these national priorities.

Merritt and Grady consider this kind of disruption of priorities that can come from giving special priority to trial participants. They do not tie this danger specifically to the issue of ancillary care. Their focus, instead, is on post-trial access to needed care. They consider the priority that might seem to fall to research participants on the basis of general considerations of reciprocity. Reciprocity is certainly a core element of the idea of justice.[9] It gets some grip on the case of research participants in roughly the same way as does the consideration of gratitude (a component of the partial-entrustment model's strength test): study participants not infrequently are willing to expose themselves to some risks and undergo some inconvenience in the furtherance of scientific research. The ideal of reciprocity lends some general support to the idea that they may be owed something in return. What Merritt and Grady (2006) persuasively argue, however, is that, if the appeal is to the general idea of reciprocity, the risk and inconvenience that the study participants have willingly undergone must be compared to the risks and inconveniences that would be suffered by whoever gets displaced by giving allocative priority to the participants. If the national system of priorities is reasonably sound and legitimate, it is likely that the

9. For confirmation of this, see, e.g., John Rawls's essay, "Justice as Reciprocity" (Rawls, 1971)—though for some corrective comment on the place of reciprocity within Rawls's mature theory of justice, see Richardson (2011).

claims of the prioritized non-participants, under general reciprocity, are at least as compelling as those of the participants.

As I would see it, this persuasive argument of Merritt and Grady's illustrates yet again—now for this special case of giving priority to research participants in the allocation of a scarce medical resource—the point that considerations of general justice are not well suited to grounding the special ancillary-care obligation. Conversely, though, claims that research participants have on account of this special obligation will defeasibly call for some departure from impartial allocation. Consider an analogous case in which such a departure is called for by a special obligation of a different sort. Suppose a doctor has promised a young mother that he will return the next week to her rural village to take another look at her baby, who is feverish with malaria. The fact of this promise will rightly put this visit higher in his priorities than it would otherwise be. It would not be acceptable, when the next week came along, for the doctor simply to reckon afresh, without taking the promise into account, how he might most effectively spend his efforts. The promise creates a special obligation that rightly alters his allocative priorities. Special ancillary-care obligations are on a par with promises in this respect. Like promissory obligations, they arise from mutually voluntary transactions between two people, setting up a morally defined relationship that makes a difference to the claims and duties of each. When such special obligations are present, we should expect justified departures from impartially just allocation. Unlike the principle of general reciprocity that Merritt and Grady explore, the special ancillary-care obligation articulates a moral claim that research participants have on the particular research team in whose study they participated. This kind of special claim will, like a promise, compete with, and resist being morally steamrollered by, considerations of impartial justice.

This resistance is defeasible. To return to the analogous case: if when the time comes for the promised repeat visit to the baby the doctor's clinic is inundated with patients in crisis, then the promise might get morally overridden by the urgent demands of the moment. Similarly, if giving priority to former research participants for access to ART really ends up taking the drugs out of the hands of poor, rural women and putting them in the hands of members of the urban, male, elite, there would be reason to question whether the ancillary-care claims of the latter group should prevail over more impartial considerations of distributive justice and respect for local political control. It would take quite a sharp clash with powerful considerations of justice wholly to override the ancillary-care obligations, however. That is partly because such conflicts will rarely be zero–sum. Research teams will tend to have sources of drugs, supplies, and trained personnel that do not entirely overlap with a host government's sources. Hence, while it is *possible* that a research team's departures from a government's priorities, in the name of respecting ancillary-care obligations, will result in a direct diversion of resources from a high-priority group to a low-priority group, it is more likely that a research team's efforts to address its ancillary-care obligations will mobilize at least some resources that would not otherwise have been available to the host nation.[10] When deliberating about conflicts between special ancillary-care claims and the demands of impartially just allocation, it may also be relevant to take into account more basic, pragmatic considerations about which alternative will best encourage the improvement of the health of those in the host nation. Once one is weighing such

---

10. See Merritt & Grady (2006) for some detailed scenarios, setting out the assumptions that would have to be met for the former, more zero–sum situation to hold. They do not claim that this situation would be typical of cases in which providing participants ancillary care might compete with national priorities.

consequences of the different alternatives, however, one's decision is no longer being ruled by justice.

I conclude, then, that honoring medical researchers' special ancillary-care obligations will not in general conflict with justice. Even if these researchers are already helping the population they are enrolling as participants, it is not unjust to recognize that they have such special obligations. The researchers laid themselves open to such special obligations in undertaking to do their work. Although undue inducement can be a concern, and should be addressed on a case-by-case basis during IRB or REC review of study protocols, provision of owed ancillary care will not in general count as unduly inducing. That is in part because providing it is morally obligatory. Justified departures from impartial justice in the allocation of medical resources is precisely what we should expect when special obligations are on the scene. Finally, research participants' special ancillary-care claims will not always prevail over other, competing moral considerations, nor does the partial-entrustment model imply that they will.[11]

## JUSTICE REINFORCING ANCILLARY-CARE CLAIMS

The negative conclusion I drew earlier in this chapter, to the effect that considerations of general justice cannot serve to ground the special ancillary-care obligation, was a narrow one. From the beginning, I have been distinguishing between this special obligation, which is what the partial-entrustment model seeks to capture, and other moral reasons why medical researchers might have obligations to provide ancillary care (see Table 1 in Chapter 1). My negative

11. See n. 10, above.

conclusion pertains only to accounting for the special ancillary-care obligation. It leaves open the possibility that considerations of justice might underwrite general ancillary-care obligations— ancillary-care obligations that do *not* specially hold as between the particular researchers and their particular research participants, as such. I turn now to a brief exploration of how this might go.

Looking at how considerations of justice might back up *general* ancillary-care obligations is well within the spirit of what Benatar and Singer have urged. Recall their criticism of approaches that focus on "micro" transactions. En route to my narrow, negative conclusion, I argued that a focus on micro transactions is just what one needs in accounting for special obligations that particular researchers owe to *their* study participants. If, however, we take this special ancillary-care obligation to be well established—whether in the way that the partial-entrustment model suggests or in some other way—then we are freed up to look around to see what other, perhaps more general considerations might be available to reinforce the special ancillary-care obligation. Considerations of general justice are prominent among these.

To see how this might go, we might focus not just on the overall account I have given of the special ancillary-care obligation but on the kinds of cases in which, according to the partial-entrustment model, participants will end up with a claim to ancillary care. As my examples have made plain, many of the strongest claims for ancillary care (assuming that the scope condition is met) will arise from participants who are dependent on the research team for care, in the sense that if the research team does not provide them the ancillary care or arrange for its provision, then they will not receive care for that disease or condition. Occasionally, this might be because the researchers are among the very few people in the world who are experts about the participants' condition. (I think, in this regard, of the impressive Host Defenses lab at the National Institutes of

Health and their ongoing natural-history studies of chronic granu-
lomatous disease.) Much more commonly, however, what accounts
for the participants' dependence on the researchers for any needed
ancillary care will be a combination of the participants' poverty, the
inadequacy of locally available medical care where they live, and
the inadequacy of their national medical insurance. In short, a high
proportion of valid special claims to ancillary care will be the claims
of the poor people living either in poor countries or in poor areas of
capitalist countries with weak national health insurance.

Considerations of general distributive justice could easily provide reasons for providing ancillary care to such people—call them
the "AC-dependent." Take, for instance, the duties of justice that
arguably arise under the heading of equality. Few now defend an
ideal of strict equality that factors down to matters as specific as
health care. Some departures from full equality, on whatever metric
is taken, seem acceptable as a matter of justice. Theorizing about
justice under the general heading of equality has lately tended to
focus on two rival sorts of position, each tolerant of some departures from literal equality: prioritarianism (e.g., Arneson, 2000;
Parfit, 1997) and sufficientarianism (e.g., Crisp, 2003; Frankfurt,
1999).[12] For our purposes here, what matters is what these two
approaches have in common, more than their differences. According
to prioritarianism, as a matter of egalitarian justice, priority should
be given to the least advantaged, who may be defined in terms of
income and wealth, in terms of "family and class origins... natural
endowments... and... fortune and luck in the course of life" (Rawls,

---

12. I set aside a line of argument that, I think, crosscuts the distinctions drawn in the text
among literal equality, prioritarianism, and sufficientarianism, namely the luck-egalitarian position (e.g., Arneson, 1989; Cohen, 1989). According to luck egalitarians,
departures from equality are justified if and only if they result from an individual's
voluntary risk-taking. In suggesting that the luck-egalitarian line of thought crosscuts
these other distinctions, I am supposing that this kind of responsibility proviso could
be attached not only to literal equality but also to priority and to sufficiency.

1999b, 83), in terms of basic capabilities (Nussbaum, 2000), or otherwise. According to sufficientarianism, what egalitarian justice instead demands is that everyone has "enough"—in the way, for example, of the *Allocative basic minimum* principle, above. In developing the conceptual contest between these two positions, philosophers have had no trouble coming up with cases in which prioritarianism and sufficientarianism would have divergent recommendations. Here, however, what matters is that these two leading rivals for how best to interpret the demands of egalitarian justice will tend to agree that the AC-dependent have claims of justice. These are people who are both among the relatively worst off in the world and among those for whom a sufficient or decent minimum standard of living has not been guaranteed.

Hence, whether by appeal to prioritarianism or to sufficientarianism, the AC-dependent can expect to be able to lean on arguments from general distributive justice. In cases such as that of the hypothetical Quinodyne, research participants may also be able to appeal to rectificatory justice to bolster their claims for ancillary care. Such claims of general distributive justice or special rectificatory justice might powerfully support ancillary-care claims. Rather than thinking of them as operating on their own, however, I suggest that we instead view them as *reinforcing* claims that the special ancillary-care obligation establishes.

Taken on their own, these arguments of distributive and rectificatory justice not only fail to generate duties specially to the participants in these researchers' studies but also fail to generate duties incumbent on researchers as such. In failing to do the latter, they lose contact with the idea of ancillary care, which is defined relative to research. To get around the general mismatch between special rectificatory justice and ancillary-care obligations, my case of Quinodyne ginned up an historical connection between the firm's resource-extraction phase and its pharmaceutical phase. This connection is admittedly very artificial. Even more to the point, however: as noted above, it still fails to establish that Quinodyne's researchers, *as researchers*, owe any reparations to the descendants of their plantation workers. If any person owes such reparations, it is the artificial and long-lived person, Quinodyne, itself. In the case of general distributive justice, it is even less clear that the researchers, *as researchers*, owe special consideration to AC-dependent participants. Assuming—what does not go without saying—that considerations of general distributive justice do generate individual duties and that some of these do fall on the researchers, they are more likely to be ones that are incumbent on them *as relatively well-off individuals* or *as people who enjoy well more than a basic minimum standard of living.*

This contact with research can be maintained, however, if we see these sorts of arguments of distributive and rectificatory justice as *reinforcing* the kind of special ancillary-care obligation set out by the partial-entrustment model. An account of these researchers' special ancillary-care obligations, such as the partial-entrustment account, can establish an obligation that falls to them as researchers and that they owe to their participants. The considerations of distributive and rectificatory justice can then come in to reinforce this special obligation. Because authors such as Benatar and Singer are so articulate about the importance of such considerations of justice in the context of international medical research, I welcome their contributions. In thinking about the grounds of ancillary-care obligations, the one proviso on which I insist is that special obligations, grounded in the "micro" transactions of particular research teams with particular research participants, must lie at the basis.

# Chapter 5

# Limits on the Waiver of Ancillary-Care Obligations

The partial-entrustment model grounds research participants' special ancillary-care claims in a special obligation that arises out of their transactions with the researchers.[1] Typically, however, claims arising out of personal transactions are waivable. If you proffer a promise of dinner out next weekend, I can take you up on the promise today and then waive my claim tomorrow, whether for selfish reasons or because I have realized that you cannot really afford to take me out to dinner. If you carelessly knock my shoes into the river, you owe me some compensation; but again, I can waive my claim to compensation. I can simply say "forget about it." Usually, potential claims of these sorts are considered waivable not only after they have concretely arisen but also in advance. Ferry operators, for instance, can tell passengers that part of the bargain in accepting passage is to take full responsibility for their personal effects, including their shoes. Similarly, operators of parking garages in common-law countries often try to disclaim any "bailment" responsibility for the vehicles in their garage, thus at least attempting to annul any claim the vehicles' owners would have that the garage get

---

1. A special claim that B has on A is the correlative (the other side of the coin) of the special obligation that A owes to B. For example, if A owes reparations to B then B has a special claim on A for those reparations.

their vehicles to safety were, say, a fire to break out.[2] If participants' special claims to ancillary care were waivable in advance in this way, then when research subjects enrolled in a study, they could simply be asked to waive in advance any ancillary-care claims that might arise. Such a practice would largely vitiate any practical implications of the approach taken here. To explain why this is not a significant worry about the partial-entrustment model, we need to examine the moral constraints on waiving claims to ancillary care.

Do we have any rights that are unwaivable, in the strong sense that their holders lack the ability—the "moral power"[3]—to waive them? The question is debated. The right not to be enslaved is often held up as the star case of a right that seems unwaivable in this sense. Intuitively, this seems to be because to enslave someone is to wrong that person so deeply—in a way so injurious to his or her moral personhood—that no one has the power to release another from the obligation not to enslave him or her. When dealing with claims to ancillary care, however, we are within the contrasting rubric of claims to positive performances. It is harder to make a compelling case that claim-rights to others' positive performances are unwaivable in this sense. I will not attempt to make such a case.[4] Instead, my argument in this chapter will be that it is harder to annul these claims than one might think and that it is generally wrong for researchers to ask participants to waive their ancillary-care claims in advance. In other words, the moral limits on waiver do not lie in the participants' lacking the moral power to waive

2. See Richardson & Belsky (2004), p. 27, analogizing bailment to the partial entrustment involved in the special ancillary-care obligation. As I indicated at 39n, however, Chapter 3's account of the basis of special ancillary-care obligations supersedes any appeal to bailment.
3. A moral power is an ability to change a person's moral claims or permissions, or lack thereof, including one's own, by one's voluntary action. Cf. Raz (1972).
4. I had attempted to make such a case in earlier versions of some of this material, some of which is effectively responded to by Wertheimer (2011, 280–282).

these claims (whether in advance or later) but in certain moral constraints on how it is possible to annul the corresponding obligations
and on when it is permissible to solicit the waiver of these claims.
This conclusion will suffice to forestall the worry that the partial-
entrustment model allows for a wholesale waiving of these claims
that would vitiate their practical importance. I will begin with why
it is difficult to annul ancillary-care obligations.

Before heading into these arguments, however, I want to forestall a possible misunderstanding. We ought to distinguish having
a right or claim to ancillary care from lacking the right to refuse
medical treatment. The right to refuse medical treatment is a right
that treatment *not* be provided to one unless one or one's authorized
surrogate has affirmatively consented to it. We all have such a right,
except in certain emergency situations. This negative right, like the
right not to be enslaved, is a good candidate for an unwaivable right.
We must remember that, whatever happens with rights to ancillary
care, this right to refuse treatment will persist. Having a claim-right
to ancillary care no more implies that one is liable to having ancillary
care forced down one's throat than having a claim-right to driving
your car on the public roads implies that you have to go anywhere.
Whenever researchers provide ancillary care or even facilitate it by
means of assisted referrals, they always ought first to check with the
individuals who need it to see if they want the care in question.

## THE DIFFICULTY OF ANNULLING
## ANCILLARY-CARE CLAIMS

Having difficulty annulling someone's obligation to provide
you ancillary care, then, by no means implies that you are liable
to having care forced on you; rather, it means that the other's
ancillary-care obligations to you are harder for you to extinguish

than are some other sorts of special obligations to you. But why is this so? The answer lies in the root of these obligations, as these were explained in Chapter 3. There, I argued that medical researchers' special ancillary-care obligations are an example of privacy-based moral entanglements. This argument rested importantly on the thought that when one (partially) waives one's *privacy* rights, what is morally going on cannot fully be understood as the giving of a special permission. In addition—I argued—one is transferring some responsibility to the person who requested the waiver. My analogy was to lending your car to a friend: In borrowing your car, your friend accrues not only special permission to drive it but also some special responsibilities to look after the car. Similarly, in accepting access to the participants' bodies and medical histories, researchers accrue not only permission for access but also some special responsibilities to look after issues they discover in acting on these permissions. In both sorts of case, I suggested, the initial waiving of rights should be viewed not as a mere permission-giving event, but also as a responsibility-transferring event. Keeping this in mind, the question in the case of special ancillary-care obligations then becomes what it takes to undo or block these moral effects of the initial waiver of privacy—which is, according to the partial-entrustment model, the crucial event in the background of all special claims to ancillary care.

Consider first what it might take to undo or annul these moral effects after the fact. In the case of lending a car to a friend, this might not be so difficult. Your friend has only to return the car and the responsibilities for dealing with it become wholly your own again. To be sure, if your friend noticed that the brake pedal was very soft or that the engine was burning oil, he should tell you about these conditions. Once he had discharged these duties of warning, however, things would be back to the initial situation. In the case of medical researchers' ancillary-care obligations, the moral *status quo ante* is not so easy to restore. That is partly because, in the vast majority of cases, the researchers will have a theoretical ability to understand the health information and a practical ability to determine how to respond to it that are vastly superior to those of the participant whose health is at stake. It is also because learning about the ancillary-care need is an irreversible event: The researchers cannot just forget about it at will. A car can be given back; not so this information. A special responsibility having been transferred to the researchers when the researcher–participant relationship was initiated, the researchers cannot divest themselves of that responsibility simply by means of a warning, either. Because of the predictably vast asymmetry in the parties' understanding, it will not do, say, simply to tell a participant, "you have stage IIB cervical cancer" or "your bilirubin levels are elevated, suggesting some challenge to your liver functions." The participant will rightly want to know what this information *means*. And starting to spell out what this information means in a way that a non-physician participant can understand will inevitably require the researcher to indicate something about what can and should be done in response to this information. But to talk to the participant about such things is to take the first steps of providing care to the participant for the disease or condition that has been discovered.

The reader may object that I already gave a case in which someone effectively waived an ancillary-care claim after a need had arisen, namely that of myself as a participant in a functional brain-scan study. "That's OK, I can take it from here," I imagined myself saying. I agree that this is a case in which *ex post* waiver of ancillary-care claims (waiver thereof after the specific need has arisen) would be effective. Part of this story about myself, however, was that my statement was presumed to be *true*. In turn, part of the assumed background that this presumption carried along with it is that I am well insured and have good access to medical professionals.

In short, I am (for the purposes of this hypothetical, certainly) the opposite of someone who is AC-dependent. Because of this, this statement effectively does more than merely renounce my claim to ancillary care—the way I might renounce my claim to compensation for my shoes, now floating down the river. It also credibly asserts that the responsibility for caring for the newly discovered condition, which otherwise would fall to the researchers, has been or will be satisfactorily placed in the capable hands of other physicians. It will be a rare thing for those with ancillary-care claims to be able truthfully or even credibly to say any such thing. (In part, this is because non-dependence on ancillary care will weaken the strength of any potential claim to it: Those with valid ancillary-care claims will tend to be more dependent on ancillary care.) Hence, the case of my probably effective *ex post* waiver serves in fact to suggest that in the contrasting cases things would be quite otherwise: These are the cases in which the responsibilities for the needed care are *not* well settled on someone else's shoulders. Attending to this complementary and presumably much more common case suggests that research participants cannot relieve the researchers of these responsibilities simply by saying *ex post* that they renounce their special ancillary-care claims.

Turn now to the possibility of anticipatory or *ex ante* waivers of ancillary-care claims. Prospective participants could be asked in advance to waive any claims to ancillary care when they signed up for a trial and to relieve the researchers of any special ancillary-care responsibilities. If these statements could be effective in both these respects, they would forestall the placement of any special ancillary-care responsibility in the hands of the researchers. I again grant that the prospective participants could waive or renounce their claims. The question is whether they can also relieve the researchers of the special responsibilities that underlie and explain their special ancillary-care obligations just by saying that they do. There are reasons to doubt it. Things would be different if the special ancillary-care claims rested on the participants' having reasonable expectations that the researchers will help them. If that were the basis of their claims, then an initial, explicit act of disclaiming would block the relevant expectations, preventing any such claims from arising. The partial-entrustment account of these claims, however, does not rest them on anyone's expectations. Instead, it rests them on the participants' having relaxed or waived their privacy rights in order to allow the researchers to gather information. Against that backdrop, what we have to ask is whether the participants can do anything that allows researchers to gather information in this way without accruing the responsibilities that would otherwise automatically come with voluntarily entering into the participants' private matters.

To probe this question, let us again consider a couple of parallel cases from outside the context of medical research. Returning to the case of The Tax Accountant and the Gambling Addict from Chapter 3, suppose that the client had said, "Look, my life is as messy as the next person's, and I'm not saying it would not be your business to worry about odd patterns of behavior that my financial transactions reveal, but I really don't want you to feel any special responsibility to help me with any such problems that you may discover in going over my taxes." Note, first of all, what an unusual statement this would be. Although I have attempted to phrase the statement idiomatically, this is hardly a boilerplate way of carrying out a standard speech act of absolving someone from responsibility, like "I forgive you." It is not easy to imagine what a "standard form" absolution would sound like in this situation. Secondly, the fact that we can and should generally assume that voluntary transactions occur between two autonomous people has complex implications, here.[5] At one level, one could say that this statement is simply reinforcing this assumption. Yet this assumption is both widespread enough and deeply enough normatively rooted that we are forced to question why something like this needs to be said. The accountant might reasonably think that the client's denial that he was warning the client about minding his own business was insincere, and so conclude that the client really was warning him to mind his own business. Equally plausibly, however, the accountant might take this overall statement as a cry for help. Psychologically, despite this attempted absolution, the accountant is still likely to feel some special responsibility towards the client once he notices the gambling addiction. Normatively, why should this attempted absolution make any difference to that? It is not *the client's* business to determine what the accountant is or is not responsible for. The independence of the accountant's judgment on this kind of issue is a hallmark of being a professional. Indeed, if Immanuel Kant is to be believed (*sapere aude!*), such independence of judgment is, more generally, a hallmark of being a mature moral agent.

Here is another case:

> *N's Seatmate's Pills:* N, a former nurse, is on the aisle on a 14-hour overnight flight to Australia. He notices that the woman next to him at the window seat is nervously fumbling with a large, segmented pill case and taking lots of the pills. Although he does not mean to butt in, he is naturally curious about why she is so anxious. As innocuously as he can, he asks her about it, excusing his remark by mentioning that he used to be a nurse. "Yes," she says. "Now, I don't want you to feel like you have to do anything about this, but since you've asked: The reason I'm so anxious is that if I can't wake myself up once every three

5. I am grateful to Leif Wenar for pressing me on this question.

hours to take my pills, I'm sure I'll have another seizure from my aneurysm by the end of the flight." Glancing again at the pills to see what they are, N judges this to be a reasonable worry.

Here again, it seems that the attempt to disclaim being the object of the other's special responsibility is both psychologically and morally ineffective. Despite the woman's attempted disclaimer, N has here gotten morally entangled in a special responsibility. Perhaps he can discharge it by lending his seatmate his alarm watch; but perhaps he will need to work out a protocol that involves waking himself up at intervals, too.

To be sure, ancillary-care obligations in the context of medical research typically arise in situations considerably different from the two cases just mentioned in important respects. In the ancillary-care cases that fall most squarely under the partial-entrustment rationale, the most salient difference will be that the participants are not yet aware of their needs for ancillary care when they sign up for the study. This difference, however, cuts two ways. It does mean that, unlike N's seatmate, such participants are not in the position of handing over to another what they know is a portentous secret.[6] By the same token, however, it means that these participants are not in a position to know what specific responsibilities they are attempting to disclaim. To put it mildly, it is awkward to attempt to absolve someone of responsibility for one-knows-not-what. "I recognize that, by carrying out study procedures, you may discover that I have medical problems of which I am now unaware. I hereby

6. Of course, study participants *can* be in this position. For instance, they may already know that they are HIV positive and yet not be suffering any symptoms that would make this seem apparent to the naked eye. My point in the text is that the partial-entrustment account does not apply as squarely to such conditions, of which the participants are already aware, as it does to conditions that are initially diagnosed by carrying out study procedures. I will explore this distinction more fully in Chapter 7.

renounce any claim for ancillary care for those problems, whatever they may turn out to be, and absolve you, the researchers, from any moral responsibility for dealing with them, whatever they are." We have all seen such absolving language in the fine print of documents cooked up by lawyers; however, it is hard to take it seriously as a moral matter. Again, the seriousness of the potential ancillary-care problems is unknown in advance. Since they potentially threaten the participants' fragile autonomy, they could be quite serious. On account of this, it seems almost as difficult for the participants anticipatorily to absolve the researchers from moral responsibility for dealing with the problems as it is for N's seatmate fully to absolve him of responsibility in the face of a problem known to be somewhat serious.[7]

The fact that special ancillary-care obligations are not fully subject to the parties' intentional shaping, whether *ex ante* or *ex post*, should not surprise us. On the defense of the partial-entrustment account elaborated in Chapter 3, these obligations arise from moral entanglements, which are, by definition, obligations that arise as unintended byproducts of mutually voluntary transactions. They have at the core, in other words, an aspect that escapes intentional management. This core is tied to what is revealed by private matters intentionally opened to inspection. Once that inspection has taken place, even if the research participants renounce the claims arising from this transaction, the transferred moral responsibility that underlies those claims will remain. It is not easily subject

7. The potential seriousness of ancillary-care problems marks a contrast with cases such as loaning someone a car. Although the risks posed to vehicles can be monetarily significant, they do not typically threaten the owner's sense of his or her practical identity. For this reason, the transfer of responsibility that typically occurs when one loans someone one's car, described in Chapter 3, will be easier to annul than the transfers of responsibility that accompany the acceptance of research participants' privacy waivers. This argument for the conclusion that it is difficult to waive or annul ancillary-care claims may draw objections on grounds of paternalism. I address the issue of paternalism in Chapter 8. I am grateful to Leif Wenar for discussion of these issues.

to intentional limitation or annulment. This suggests that even if participants were *ex ante* to renounce any potential claims to ancillary care, the researchers would retain some moral responsibility to provide it.

## MORAL CONSTRAINTS ON SOLICITING WAIVERS OF ANCILLARY-CARE CLAIMS

In the last section, I argued that it is difficult for research participants to annul researchers' ancillary-care obligations by waiving or attempting to waive claims to ancillary care. Even if it were fully possible for participants to do so, however, it would often be wrong for researchers to solicit waivers of ancillary-care claims from their participants. Wertheimer (2011, 282), after arguing that ancillary-care claims are waivable, says the following: "To be clear, I do not claim to have shown that investigators should be permitted to ask prospective subjects to waive a right to ancillary care if they have such right." To this further issue of the permissibility of soliciting waivers of ancillary-care claims we must now turn. Here I want to highlight two different kinds of reason why doing so will often be impermissible, one grounded in quite general facts about those with the strongest claims to ancillary care and another grounded in the features of ancillary-care obligations emphasized by the partial-entrustment account.

The first of these sorts of reason builds on the considerations of justice developed in the previous chapter. There, I noted in a general way that those with the strongest claims to ancillary care will tend to be the AC-dependent. In addition, I argued, people dependent on researchers for access to medical care will typically be people who are at least suffering from the effects of past injustices, if not also from ongoing injustice. My general conclusion about this in the previous chapter was that, for this reason, considerations of distributive and rectificatory justice will tend to reinforce ancillary-care claims. One way this reinforcement will work is by generating moral limits on asking potential participants to waive their claims to ancillary care. As Benatar and Singer have remarked, "attempting to achieve a closer and more direct linkage between health research and healthcare services is the least that privileged researchers can do to alleviate the plight of people in poor countries" (Benatar & Singer, 2010, 195). And, we might add, the plight of the underinsured poor in inner cities and rural areas in developed countries. Admittedly, not *all* medical researchers will count as "privileged" in the relevant sense. Bit by bit, developing countries are building up their own capacities to conduct medical research. An observational study of cryptosporidial diarrhea carried out in Ethiopia by an entirely Ethiopian team of parasitologists funded by the Ethiopian government, for instance, would not well exemplify the idea of research being carried out by "privileged researchers." This qualification aside, however, it remains true that most medical research is sponsored by the governments of the industrialized countries or by the world's giant pharmaceutical corporations and includes researchers from these countries on each study's team of investigators. Justice calls for giving priority to the poor and oppressed. Providing them ancillary care is one good way that researchers, as researchers, can give them priority. Hence, in most studies enrolling poor participants, considerations of justice will stand as reasons why researchers ought not to ask their participants anticipatorily to waive their ancillary-care claims.[8]

---

8. While loyalty to the aims of science does serve as a justifiable basis for limiting the ancillary care provided even to the poorest and most oppressed, that consideration already figures into the partial-entrustment model's test of strength and should not be double-counted in determining whether it is wrong to ask participants to waive their ancillary-care claims.

The second reason why it will generally be wrong for medical researchers to ask their participants anticipatorily to waive their ancillary-care claims connects with the basis of these claims in waivers of privacy rights, as set out in Chapter 3. It also builds on the point, developed in the previous section, that it is difficult for researchers to shuck off the special responsibilities that underlie their ancillary-care obligations.

My account of these underlying responsibilities was developed in Chapter 3. There, in developing an account of how accepting someone's waivers of privacy can get one morally entangled in ancillary-care obligations, I argued that when rights are waived, responsibilities are often transferred that have to do with the underlying purpose of the rights. In the case of privacy rights, I argued, this purpose is crucially connected with protecting the individual's fragile capacity of autonomy, especially insofar as it depends on the individual's confidence in his or her ability to make up his or her mind. Privacy rights tend to attach to items the public exposure of which might threaten this confidence. Sharing information on such matters puts an individual in a potentially awkward situation in which, under the unaccustomed gaze of another, he or she must decide how to go on.

Connect this, now, to the individual who is invited anticipatorily to waive his or her ancillary-care claims. Let us again concentrate, as we did at the end of the previous section, on individuals as yet unaware of their needs for ancillary care. This means that we are talking about an unexpected diagnosis. As we saw in Chapter 3, the general duty to warn will in any case require that the researchers communicate this diagnosis to the participant.[9] Assuming that the

---

9. The duty to rescue, of which the duty to warn is a special case, being a general duty, waiver of a claim to rescue seems generally to be irrelevant or impossible. Suppose someone posts a suicide note at the entrance to a bridge, indicating that he waives his right to rescue. Should he still be alive when he hits the water below, this note would not nullify

researchers comply with this moral requirement and do communicate this diagnosis, the participant will be faced with having to assimilate an unexpected diagnosis into his or her self-conception. Insofar as the diagnosis is a serious one or involves threats to capabilities that the person cares a lot about (as a musician cares about finger dexterity, for instance), the necessary psychological adjustment will be a difficult one, one that may well leave the individual feeling at the mercy of forces beyond his or her control. But helping the individual participant cope with such challenges is precisely the kind of special responsibility that, by accepting the person's privacy waivers, the researcher has, in a partial way, taken on. The researchers' best way of discharging this responsibility, we have been supposing, is to provide or arrange for medical care that helps the individual fight off this potential challenge to feeling that he or she can go on with deciding how to live. These facts thus provide a basis for arguing that it is likely to be wrong for medical researchers to ask their participants anticipatorily to waive their claims to ancillary care.

In thus explaining why it is generally wrong for researchers to ask research participants to waive in advance their ancillary-care claims, the idea of entrustment built into the partial-entrustment model is central. It is the transfer of underlying responsibilities, as I argued in Chapter 3, that creates an implicit entrustment. This transfer of responsibilities arises from the participants' partial waivers of their privacy rights. In the present discussion of whether the participants might also be asked to waive their ancillary-care

---

a passerby's (perhaps non-directed) duty to rescue him. Those who ski past a ski area's boundary signs spelling out in giant letters that off-piste skiing is forbidden might be taken to waive their claim-rights to rescue, if such directed claim-rights exist; but they do not thereby nullify the ski area's general (and perhaps non-directed) duty to rescue them (although they do certainly undertake a liability to bearing the expenses of any rescue). Generally speaking, then, waiver of claims to rescue (including claims to warning) seems to be, if not impossible, at least ineffectual in nullifying duties to rescue.

claims, there is no talk of the participants revoking or in any way taking back their privacy waivers. The privacy waivers relevant to setting the scope of the special ancillary-care obligation are the ones that the researchers need in order to proceed with their study without violating the participants' privacy rights. In contemplating potential ancillary-care claims arising, we are imagining that, by acting on these privacy waivers, the researchers have discovered medical needs in their participants. This means that we are supposing not only that the privacy waivers are not revoked but also that they are relevantly acted on by the researchers. The work that the idea of entrustment does, here, is to help us understand how, independently of whether or not participants also waive their claims to ancillary care, the researchers retain a special responsibility to concern themselves with protecting their participants' fragile autonomy. As Chapter 3 argued, this special responsibility *supports* special claims to ancillary care by providing a focus for specifying the general duty of beneficence. This special responsibility neither *entails* special claims to ancillary care nor is it the flip side of special ancillary-care obligations. As such, whether this special responsibility that is entrusted to researchers when participants enroll in studies persists is conceptually independent of whether the participants waive their claims to ancillary care. This means that we may appeal to this special responsibility in assessing the moral limits on asking participants to waive these claims without assuming the conclusion.

What argument can be given for the desired conclusion? Let me now try to assemble pieces into such an argument. I will begin by stating a principle of restraint. This principle articulates the moral basis for limiting the advance solicitation of rights waivers. As applied to ancillary-care issues, this principle is in the first instance a limitation on the actions of the researchers. Nonetheless, limiting what the researchers may permissibly do indirectly limits the options that participants will face. Accordingly, I have framed the principle in such a way that it skirts potential objections about paternalistically limiting the participants' liberties in the name of protecting them. It does so by framing things so that any limitation on the participants' liberty that is indirectly involved is one that could be grounded in what those individuals would want were they fully informed. As such, any paternalism that might be thought to be involved would in any case count as what is known as "soft" paternalism, which is widely conceded to be unobjectionable (cf. Feinberg, 1971; Feinberg, 1986). The principle of restraint in question is the following:

(1) *Principle of Restraint in Soliciting Rights Waivers:* It is wrong to solicit waivers of claim-rights from people where one has (a) significantly superior knowledge of the risks involved, (b) strong reason to believe that these people lack an adequate basis for determining whether they could cope with these claims going unfulfilled, and (c) some special reason to care about whether they can cope with these claims going unfulfilled.

I have recently reminded you that clause (a) is almost always fulfilled in the case we are talking about. Hence, we can say:

(2) Medical researchers generally have significantly superior knowledge of the ancillary-care risks facing their study participants than their study participants do.

What about the other conditions of the principle?

The next steps of the argument are mainly empirical ones offered in support of the claim that study participants generally satisfy this principle's condition (b):

(3) Study participants will generally lack an adequate basis for anticipating what diagnoses their participation in a study would reveal.

(4) Unexpected diagnoses, at least when they concern serious illnesses or threatening conditions, threaten also to destabilize the right-holder's self-conception.

(5) It is difficult to know in advance how well one would be able to cope with a threat to the stability of one's self-conception, especially if one does not receive help in addressing the threat.

(6) Hence, since study participants are not in a position to anticipate what potentially destabilizing diagnoses they might face nor how well they could cope with these in the absence of material help therewith, there is strong reason to believe that they typically lack an adequate basis for determining whether they could cope with their ancillary-care claims going unfulfilled.

Next, in support of the claim that trial participants typically satisfy principle (1)'s condition (c), and drawing on the argument of the previous section, we have:

(7) Medical researchers generally have a responsibility, difficult to annul, to look out for their study participants' autonomy, and specifically their fragile human capacity to make up their own minds.

(8) A threat to one's self-conception of the kind mentioned in (3) is a threat to one's fragile human capacity to make up one's own mind.

(9) Hence, medical researchers generally have a non-annullable responsibility (and *a fortiori*, a special reason) to care about whether their research participants could cope with their ancillary-care claims going unfulfilled.

Therefore, since claims to ancillary care in the context of medical research will paradigmatically involve new medical diagnoses, we can conclude by appeal to the above principle of restraint that it is generally wrong for medical researchers to solicit waivers of ancillary-care claims.

This conclusion is a hedged one. As I noted in Chapter 3, some particular ancillary-care needs will involve more potential threat to an individual participant's autonomy than will others. The argument could be made more definite and nuanced by distinguishing among different candidate diagnoses in terms of their likely effect in destabilizing individuals' self-conceptions. The argument will not, for instance, have any strong implications for the behavior of researchers who discover, in the course of their study of the effect of sexually transmitted diseases on HIV transmission, that some of their female participants have yeast infections (vaginal candidiasis). Still, there will be a rough correlation between the most difficult and expensive courses of ancillary care and those occasions for ancillary care that are most threatening to the stability of a participant's self-conception. Accordingly, the argument suffices to defend a very significant moral limit on the advance collection of waivers of ancillary-care claims.

Nothing in the argument of this section implies that it would be morally wrong or impossible for prospective participants in medical research to *proffer* (unsolicited) waivers of their ancillary-care claims.[10] Perhaps, as a way to lure medical researchers to their district, a district's residents might even get together and collectively—indeed, unanimously—decide to trumpet the fact that they welcome researchers who proceed without providing any ancillary care. In so doing, they would each be taking some risk with regard to their ability to cope without ancillary care. On this account, their

10. Again, I am grateful to Leif Wenar for raising this point.

LIMITS ON WAIVER OF ANCILLARY-CARE OBLIGATIONS

initiative might well be misguided. Nonetheless, their action would not run afoul of the principle of restraint, which is narrowly stated as a limitation on the *solicitation* of waivers of ancillary-care claims. I do think that, in responding to some poor district of Mali or Haiti that had put together such an enticement to researchers, those responsible for selecting their research sites would face delicate questions about whether it is permissible to take advantage of such an offer. Arguably, the principle of restraint should be broadened so as to cover not only soliciting waivers of ancillary-care claims but also to responding to proffers of such waivers. As a practical matter, however, it is simpler to recur to considerations of justice. Among the most delicate questions raised by proffered waivers of ancillary-care claims will be ones having to do with the broader issues of distributive and rectificatory justice that were discussed in Chapter 4 and that have already come up in this chapter. Suppose that a group of researchers working on extremely drug-resistant (XDR) tuberculosis would not be able to afford to do their study in such a poor district, so terribly lacking in health infrastructure, if they had to provide ancillary care, but that without having to do so, they could afford it. It is possible that by choosing to do their research in such a district, they would be doing the people of the district a favor, at least by giving them temporary access to some non-ancillary medical care—perhaps more medical care than they otherwise would have had—and by doing something to boost the local economy. It is also possible, however, that in choosing to locate their research in such a district while not providing ancillary care that would otherwise be obligatory, these researchers would be criticizably taking advantage of the injustices that have put these people in such difficult straits.[11] I have not chosen the example of such impoverished

11. Indeed, what would make many such decisions difficult is the fact that these two possibilities are mutually compatible.

districts arbitrarily: It is precisely such areas that are most likely to be desperate enough to lure medical researchers that they would consider waiving their ancillary-care claims as a way to do so. Hence, while legitimately accepting a community's proffered waiver of ancillary-care obligations is a theoretical possibility, the opportunities to do so permissibly would be sharply limited by considerations of justice.

I conclude that since it is very difficult to annul the special responsibility underlying medical researchers' ancillary-care obligations and generally wrong for medical researchers to solicit advance waivers of their participants' ancillary-care claims, the partial-entrustment model robustly resists the threat that waiver might vitiate its practical implications.

Chapter 6

# Gradations of Ancillary-Care Responsibility

It is now widely accepted that researchers testing new treatments for HIV-AIDS have some moral responsibility to insure that the treatment remains "reasonably available" to participants after the study is over (CIOMS, 2002 guideline 21).[1] Providing preventative and post-trial treatment to participants in HIV prevention trials has also been discussed (e.g., WHO/UNAIDS, 2004; MacQueen et al. 2003; Barsdorf et al. 2010). But what about clinical or epidemiological researchers conducting *non-HIV* research in developing countries who encounter participants with HIV-AIDS, for whom any HIV-AIDS care would clearly count as ancillary care? While the efforts of such programs as PEPFAR and the Global Fund have helped make antiretroviral treatment (ART) more widely available in developing countries, and although the picture is changing fast on the ground, we remain a long way from the day when we can say that ART is available to anyone who needs it (Bennett & Chanfreau, 2005; McGough et al., 2005; Treatment Action Campaign, 2008). For example, in mid-2010, due to a shortage of government funds, Uganda was facing an acute shortage of antiretrovirals (Wasswa, 2010). Where ART is not readily

1. This chapter is adapted from Richardson (2007). Originally published in *American Journal of Public Health* (97) 11; Nov 2007: 1956–1961. Reprinted with permission.

available, what obligations, if any, do researchers in non-HIV trials have to ensure that these participants get ART? If those who sponsor and carry out medical research have a responsibility to provide ART to trial participants, this can be conceived as an obligation to take the steps necessary to increase the overall availability of ART and skilled personnel in the country or countries hosting the research, if only for the benefit of their trial participants. By so conceiving it, we may sidestep the difficult issues of justice that would arise if trial participants were to be seen as competing with their co-nationals for priority in access to a fixed supply of anti-retrovirals or medical professionals: These issues of justice were addressed in Chapter 4.

Here I would like to use these difficult questions about addressing HIV-AIDS as a matter of ancillary care in order to illustrate two important steps in bringing the partial-entrustment model to bear in practice: (1) how the partial-entrustment model's test of scope can be elaborated to reflect important variations in study design and (2) how the model's test of strength can be systematically applied without presuming spurious ways of commensurating the sub-dimensions relevant to a given claim's strength.[2] The strength test is obviously sensitive to contextual variations; the idea of scope is more sensitive thereto than one might think. Putting these two facts together implies that the model is capable of generating quite a range of verdicts as to the stringency of ancillary-care obligations of a given kind with respect to a given study.

One reason it makes sense to look for gradations in the stringency in ancillary-care obligations is well illustrated by the many gradations of possible response there are to the needs of HIV-AIDS

---

2. For an analysis that takes advantage of the partial-entrustment model's ability to capture variations in the strength of ancillary-care obligations, as these arise in the very different context of genomic research, see Beskow & Burke (2010).

sufferers in a developing country. For them, researchers might provide any of the following levels of care (Tucker & Slack, 2004):

- recommend treatment and provide a referral
- provide only palliative care for opportunistic infections
- provide palliative care and try to arrange funds to pay for ART
- provide palliative care and provide or pay for ART
- provide palliative care, ART, and monitoring

With regard to each of these levels of care, there is also the question of how long it is to be provided: Just for the duration of the trial? After the trial is over, as well? For the participant's lifetime? Given this wide range of possible responses, there is no reason to think of researchers' responsibilities towards HIV-AIDS sufferers in all-or-nothing terms.

Recall that the partial-entrustment model of the special ancillary-care obligation has a two-pronged structure. According to its first, scope test, it is the permissions researchers had to have obtained to do the study permissibly that determine which aspects of a participant's health are within the *scope* of their special ancillary-care obligations. That a disease or condition falls within the scope of the researchers' special ancillary-care responsibility, however, does not according to the model settle whether they ought to provide care for it. To settle this further question, one must also take up the model's second prong and assess the strength of the participants' claim to care. The model's five strength factors, as set out in Chapter 2, are the following:

- participants' vulnerability (how badly off they would be if they did not receive help)
- participants' degree of dependence on the researchers (whether they lack other sources of possible help)

- participants' uncompensated risks or burdens
- the expectable depth (intensity and duration) of the researcher–participant relationship
- the cost to the researchers (in money, personnel, and study power) of providing the relevant care

To simplify the present discussion of gradations in researchers' special ancillary-care responsibilities, as these arise regarding HIV-AIDS among research participants in developing countries, we should focus on those factors that will show the biggest variance from trial to trial. HIV-AIDS sufferers, who do poorly without help, are all terribly vulnerable. Their dependence on researchers for access to HIV-AIDS care seems likely to vary more from country to country than from trial to trial. What will importantly vary, among studies in which HIV-AIDS is likely to arise as an ancillary-care need, are the depth of the researcher–participant relationship and the cost of providing a given level of care.

To preview the kinds of case in which these issues of detail and nuance will arise, let me describe a real case. A recent study of the effect of nitazoxanide on Zambian children with cryptosporidiosis exemplifies how HIV-AIDS care might arise as an ancillary-care obligation (Amadi et al., 2002). This trial enrolled 50 HIV-seropositive and 50 HIV-seronegative children, all suffering from cryptosporidial diarrhea. It concluded that while nitazoxanide significantly reduced mortality and morbidity in the children uninfected with HIV, it was not effective in those who were HIV seropositive. In this case, HIV-AIDS care would count as ancillary care: HIV-AIDS care, at any of the levels distinguished above, was required neither by the study's design nor by trial safety. Nonetheless, HIV-AIDS was central to how the trial was designed and conducted. Although cryptosporidiosis was the disease under study, the researchers were necessarily aware of the

HIV-AIDS needs of the 50 children whose seropositivity qualified them for the study. So this is a case in which HIV-AIDS care counts as ancillary care, and yet the fact that claims for such ancillary care satisfy of the scope requirement is obvious from even a cursory examination of the study design. I want now to suggest how the scope requirement can be elaborated to capture the significance of this fact.

## WITHIN THE SCOPE: MINIMALLY, CLEARLY, OR CENTRALLY?

There is no need to treat the question of whether a given aspect of the participants' health is within the scope of the researchers' special ancillary-care responsibility as a binary, all-or-nothing matter. In the Zambian nitazoxanide trial, participants' HIV-AIDS was *clearly* within the scope of what has been entrusted to them, as the trial design called for stratifying the participants on the basis of their HIV status. Many studies involve HIV-related permissions more minimally—for example, those that simply request potential participants' permission to screen for seropositivity, where that is an exclusion criterion. By contrast, some studies that are not HIV-AIDS treatment trials focus on HIV-AIDS even more centrally than do studies that stratify by HIV status. Examples of the last sort include maternal–fetal transmission studies, HIV vaccine trials, and comorbidity studies. The widely discussed case of HIV-prevention trials is thus accommodated within the present analysis. In a given study, then, HIV-AIDS may be:

- *minimally within scope:* for example, if HIV-AIDS status is an exclusion criterion or is encountered in an unpredictable way by carrying out study procedures

- *clearly within scope:* for example, if HIV-AIDS status is important to the study design but is not a study endpoint
- *centrally within scope:* for example, if the study endpoints include aspects of HIV-AIDS, whether seropositivity, morbidity, or mortality

In all three of these variants, HIV-AIDS care is within the scope of what is entrusted to the researchers by the permissions participants give during the informed-consent process. What the scope gradations reflect, here, are variations in how firmly this fact is embedded in the study's design.

While I hope these gradations of scope, as just presented, are clear enough in their own terms, it would be reassuring for the HIV-AIDS context to have a more general, principled basis for them. To apply these gradations more generally to other types of ancillary-care needs and other types of medical research, such a principled basis is necessary. So that I may begin to set one out, let me go through these gradations again, this time more abstractly. I suggest that we think of them by reference to how radically the research plan would have to be changed in order for a given finding no longer to fall within the scope of entrustment. The notion of the radicalness of a possible change in the research plan may, in turn, be understood by reference to the presumptive aim of the plan and the ways it arranges means to that (intermediate) end. Consider again an observational study of the transplacental transmission of malaria. In abstract terms, the presumptive aim of such a study is:

(1) to find out more about transplacental transmission of malaria

In addition, we can already tell from the context—for we are talking about medical research involving human subjects—that these scientists aim to find out more in a certain way: not by doing a study in other animals or by doing biochemical modeling of the conditions in the placenta, but by observing mothers and their babies. Hence, a second layer of description of the study's aim is the following:

(2) to find out more about transplacental transmission of malaria by observing mothers and their babies

Call this the study's "core aim." More specifically, these researchers will look to see how many of the babies end up infected with malaria. This study endpoint is thus built in to the first layer of means associated with the study's core aim. We might naturally combine it with that core aim, to get the following:

(2′) to study the transplacental transmission of malaria by observing the rate of malaria infection in the babies of pregnant women infected with malaria

Now suppose that this same study also stratified its participants according to whether they are also suffering from schistosomiasis. In relation to the same core aim, this would be a means of secondary importance. That is because although one can observationally find out about transplacental malaria transmission without stratifying by schistosomiasis, one cannot observationally find out about transplacental malaria transmission without observing the rate of malarial infection in the babies. Thus we arrive at a hypothetical study design, hierarchically arranged as follows:

(3) to study the transplacental transmission of malaria by observing the rate of malaria infection in the babies of pregnant women infected with malaria, recording data about this rate in a way that stratifies the participants in terms of whether they are also suffering from schistosomiasis

Fourth and finally, in relation to any such proposed study design, there will be questions about how to carry it out in a way that is safe or that is likely to generate significant results. Safety and soundness are requirements of any legitimate study involving human subjects, and as such are not peculiar to the aims of any one of them. Exclusion criteria of various kinds exemplify in one way this fourth layer of elaboration of a researcher's plans. For instance, it would be possible to study the transplacental transmission of malaria by observing the rate of malaria infection in the babies of pregnant women infected with malaria (while stratifying the results on the basis of whether the mothers are also suffering from schistosomiasis) without excluding potential participants who also have drug-resistant tuberculosis; but there might be reasons why the research team could not safely handle those with drug-resistant TB (or could not safely isolate the other participants from them). If this fact about safety were, counterfactually, not to hold, then such people could be included without disrupting the researchers' plans, as stated in (3). This shows that such an exclusion criterion is even more remote from these researchers' core aim than are the other layers we have examined. Being discovered by the initial screening done to determine eligibility for study participation or in an unforeseeable way by carrying out study procedures puts a given claim for ancillary care within the scope of entrustment in a minimal way; but if a given claim's being within the scope can be deduced in advance from more central aspects of the nature of the study, then the claim is more clearly within the scope.

In relation to the gradations that the layers generated by the nested ends and means within a research team's plans, my suggested, three-tier terminology of "centrally," "clearly," and "minimally" is a heuristic simplification. As the rather fine-grained difference between (2) and (2′) illustrates, it would be difficult to establish a fully general and non-arbitrary way of counting the number of end–means layers. In relation to the widely accepted practice of setting out and reviewing scientific protocols for studies involving human subjects, however, the idea of a study's endpoints provides a highly salient and clearly relevant place to draw a line. Without looking to see whether the babies end up with malaria, one does not have much of an observational study of transplacental transmission of the disease. Hence, a participating baby's malaria is "centrally" within the scope. The stratification by reference to schistosomiasis, by contrast, can be conceptualized as a matter that pertains rather to data analysis. One will presumably have collected various other demographic and health data from the participants at the outset, and might end up variously stratifying the results, depending on what stratifications end up revealing illuminating patterns. Hence, a participant's schistosomiasis is "clearly," but not centrally, within the scope.

With these gradations in the satisfaction of the scope require-ment thus explained, I turn to the gradations in the various dimen-sions that fall under the partial-entrustment model's heading of "strength." In their case, there is no conceptual difficulty in the idea of gradation. Still, some concrete elaboration and some heu-ristic terminology will be helpful in order to handle the contextual variations among cases involving HIV-AIDS care as an ancillary matter.


## VARIATIONS IN THE EXPECTABLE DEPTH OF THE RESEARCHER–PARTICIPANT RELATIONSHIP

Variations in the depth of the relationship between researcher and participant affect the strength of ancillary-care obligations in part because the longer and more intensely one interacts with someone, the more effort one must make not to treat that person as a mere means. That concern is never nil. Still, compare:

- a long-term hospital inpatient with a life-threatening illness
- a healthy person who provides only one sputum sample or buccal swab

It takes a lot more effort to avoid treating as a mere means an inpatient whose severe illness calls for many intensive interactions.

For research-ethics purposes, as I have emphasized, it is the expectable depth of the researcher–patient relationship that matters. This should be determined on the basis of the study protocol, rather than on the basis of how things happen to turn out, which will be affected by morally irrelevant variations in individuals' psychologies. In relation to studies that touch on HIV-AIDS, the following list illustrates how the depth of the researcher–participant relationship can be expected to vary:

- *minimal depth:* studies screening out the HIV-positive; studies confined to an analysis of existing medical records
- *low depth:* studies involving only a few brief interactions with the participants
- *medium depth:* studies involving recurrent visits over a few years or intensive interactions over shorter periods
- *high depth:* studies involving frequent follow-up over a long term or involving intensive monitoring of inpatients

Maternal–fetal transmission studies are typically low depth, as they ordinarily involve only an enrollment and counseling stage, testing the mother, perhaps some monitoring during the pregnancy, and testing of the newborn. The Zambian nitazoxanide trial exemplifies a medium-depth relationship, as it involved ill children, half also HIV positive, who were each hospitalized for the 8-day duration of the study. Higher-depth studies would include those involving longer-term hospitalizations, such as studies of HIV-related diarrheal wasting among inpatients, and long-term comorbidity or vaccine studies that involve recurrent interactions with participants over many years.

## VARIATION IN RELATIVE COST

The social importance of the general goal of research makes the cost of providing ancillary care a morally relevant concern. A rough way to estimate the degree to which incurring monetary costs will frustrate scientific goals is to assess that cost relative to the relevant research budget. Similarly, the diversion of research personnel time should be assessed relative to the availability of research personnel, often a serious constraint in developing-country settings; and costs having to do with confounding results and having to drop participants from a study should be assessed in relation to the degree of difficulty of obtaining significant research results. Here, for simplicity's sake, I concentrate on the monetary costs of providing ART. I abstract from the difficulties of appropriately monitoring such treatment in places with little medical infrastructure, for while these difficulties may be overwhelming, it is difficult to predict how they will vary from study to study. Ethically, the important question about monetary cost is whether it is negligible, serious, or heavy in relation to the research budget. It is not the absolute monetary figure that matters. For purposes of comparison, I will focus on the costs of lifetime ART provision.

An example of a type of study in which the monetary costs of providing lifetime ART to participants who need it is likely to be *low* in relation to the study budget is a Phase I HIV-vaccine trial. Since Phase I trials are relatively short, it is unlikely that many of the participants will become HIV positive during the trial; yet the budgets of such studies are not very low, as quite close monitoring of participants' health is required.

A type of study in which the monetary costs of providing ART to participants who need it is likely to be *serious* in relation to the study budget is a study of late-stage comorbidities, such as diarrheal wasting. In such cases, although all of the participants may need ART, their life expectancies are so low that the total cost of providing them with lifetime ART, while appreciable, is unlikely to be very high in relation to the research budget.

Correspondingly, a type of study in which the monetary costs of providing ART to participants who need it is likely to be *heavy* in relation to the study budget is a maternal-to-child transmission (MTCT) study. Because the researcher–participant interaction in such studies is relatively low, the budgets of such studies are also likely to be relatively low. MTCT rates, however, are about 16% when nevirapine is used and significantly higher when it is not ( Jackson et al., 2003). Further, the life expectancy of the HIV-infected babies, given that they are provided with ART, will be much longer than that of adults with late-stage comorbidities. The mothers will also need ART. A relatively extreme example within this general category is provided by the observational, community-randomized study conducted in the Rakai district of Uganda from 1994 to 1999 regarding the effects of placental malaria on MTCT (Brahmbhatt et al., 2003). Because this was an observational study, it was presumably relatively cheap to conduct. The MTCT rate was relatively high in this setting, however, as nevirapine was unavailable in rural Uganda during this period.

## PUTTING THESE FACTORS TOGETHER

It would be a mistake either to expect a simple ethical calculus to resolve such difficult issues or to push for a way to quantify the analysis. The factors in play, here, are mutually incommensurable, and resist calibration along a single metric. It is often said that responsible bodies, such as IRBs or RECs, must "weigh" or "balance" such competing factors; but such talk produces only an illusion of precision (cf. Richardson, 2000). At some point, to be sure, principled guidance may run out. One may, in practice, have to fall back on one's intuitive sense of which of two factors, in a given set of circumstances, is more important. In general, however, it is desirable to extend the reach of principled guidance, whose merits people can publicly debate, postponing and limiting inevitable appeals to intuition (cf. Rawls, 1999b, 36f.). Here, I seek to illustrate how far one can get, using the factors set out above, without either falling back on such intuitive weighing or misleadingly purporting to locate a single, quantitative basis for one's decisions.

Despite remaining appropriately qualitative, this analysis does suggest some definite conclusions, allowing us in a good number of cases to compare the relative stringency of ancillary-care obligations for providing ART.

Consider the following four types of study in which HIV-AIDS care would count as ancillary care:

- *Studies that screen out the HIV-seropositive in a setting with high HIV prevalence:* In such cases, the ancillary-care obligation to provide ART to those screened out will be minimal, as these participants' HIV status is only minimally within the scope, the depth of the relationship is low, and the costs of treating them could well be very high in relation to the study budget.[3]

- *MTCT studies like the Rakai study.* While the depth of relationship remains low and the costs remain high, in the Rakai case the HIV-positive status of the mothers is an *inclusion* criterion and the HIV status of the infants is an endpoint. Hence, the principal difference between these first two cases is with regard to scope, yielding a more stringent claim on behalf of the Rakai participants.

- *Studies of HIV-related wasting among inpatients:* Compare these to the Rakai MTCT study. In both, HIV-AIDS status is central to the scope of the researchers' responsibility; but the depth of engagement will be higher in the latter and the cost in relation to the study budget will be lower. Hence, the overall case for providing ART to participants who need it is stronger in the HIV-related wasting studies.

- *A hypothetical, Phase III HIV-vaccine trial:* Compare this to HIV-related wasting studies. Again, the HIV status is central in each type of study and the depth of the researcher–participant is high in each (intense in the case of the wasting inpatients, of long duration in the case of the vaccine-trial participants). The predictable difference is in the cost of providing ART in relation to the overall study budget, which will likely be lower in the case of the vaccine trial. Accordingly, the ancillary-care obligation seems stronger in the vaccine-trial case.

---

3. For further discussion of those determined ineligible to participate in a study, see the following chapter.

Compared with trials that merely screen out the HIV-positive, the Zambian nitazoxanide trial involves a more stringent ancillary-care obligation: HIV-AIDS care is more clearly within the scope, the relationship is deeper, and the cost in relation to the study budget will not be greater. By contrast, compared to the HIV-related wasting studies, the Zambian nitazoxanide trial presents a less stringent obligation: HIV-AIDS is not centrally within the scope and the relationship is less deep. We do not have a clear basis to rank it in relation to the Rakai MTCT study, however, as the factor of scope pulls one way and the depth of relationship pulls another.

Placing all of these comparative results on a qualitative grid displays four grades of ancillary-care obligation (Fig. 4). In these examples, the two dimensions of scope and depth of relationship suffice to array the alternatives, as the factor of cost does not alter these particular rankings. Obviously, in the full range of studies, each of the factors can vary independently, making the rankings more complex. Although, for purposes of illustration, I have focused only on cases involving HIV care that is needed as

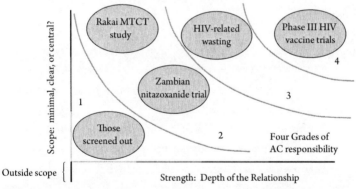

Figure 4. Four Grades of Ancillary-Care Obligation for ART Provision. Studies farther to the north and east on the graph incur a higher grade of ancillary-care obligation. Because the scales of the two axes cannot be compared, not all pairs of cases can be compared. The dimension of cost is not shown. (This figure appeared in Richardson, 2007. Reproduced with permission of Koninklijke Brill NV.)

ancillary care, nothing in this method of comparison requires that the care involved in the different studies be for the same disease or condition.

With regard to studies of HIV-related wasting and to HIV-vaccine trials, the argument explored here, which is based on the special ancillary-care obligation, should be seen as supplementing whatever arguments can be mounted on the basis of justice, the duty of rescue, or a more general beneficence (e.g., Benatar & Singer, 2000 and 2010; Shapiro & Benatar, 2005). The WHO seems to have been moving towards accepting such arguments (WHO, 2004). For these cases, the partial-entrustment model bolsters these attempts to develop the idea of the standard of care, providing some definiteness as well as a principled basis for recognizing gradations. Going beyond the range of cases on which the WHO seems to have been focusing, the model implies that some researchers who are not centrally dealing with HIV-AIDS nonetheless have some obligation to address the HIV-AIDS needs of their participants.

## CONCLUSION

A graduated conception of researchers' special ancillary-care obligations for ART provision is desirable because the range of possible responses is also graduated. The ethical analysis presented here cannot begin to indicate *which* grade of ancillary-care obligation corresponds to *which* grade of response. On the one hand, the difficulties of coordinating and monitoring ART in many settings will make that option unreasonable in many places. On the other hand, creative ways of forming partnerships to help fund ART provision or to lower drug costs may make ART provision more affordable in some contexts (Wendler, Emanuel & Lie 2004; Shapiro & Benatar, 2005). Further, in all contexts, the social effects of making ART specially available to participants must be considered, as Merritt and Grady (2006) have argued. The present analysis does not aim to settle the bottom-line question of what should be done where, but to provide research sponsors and RECs or IRBs with well-grounded, gradable, and context-sensitive factors—scope, depth of relationship, and cost in relation to research budget—they can use in determining in which cases ancillary-care considerations call for non–HIV-AIDS researchers to address the HIV-AIDS needs of their study participants. As illustrated, the analysis can generate definite, comparative results without attempting to treat the various qualitative factors in a quantitative way. It shows that the partial-entrustment model's inclusion of a test of the strength of specific ancillary-care claims does not make the model unworkable.

In the range of cases chosen for the sake of illustration, the analysis yields the conclusion that there is one type in which the case for ART provision appears particularly compelling, namely later-phase HIV-vaccine trials. The ancillary-care argument for this conclusion converges with the justice-based argument put forward by the HIV Vaccine Trials Network and others (Barsdorf et al., 2010; Fitzgerald et al., 2003; Shaffer et al., 2006). For other types of trial, in which HIV-AIDS is less central to the study design, the question of providing HIV-AIDS treatment as ancillary care will prove more challenging. Nonetheless, as this chapter's analysis shows, the partial-entrustment model's two-pronged approach provides IRBs and RECs with a workable basis for analyzing and prioritizing these other claims, as well.

Chapter 7

# Issues for Further Exploration

The previous chapter illustrated how the partial-entrustment model can be put to use in practice in a context-sensitive yet principled way. The examples I considered there all involved research in developing countries on diseases prevalent there, which is but one of many different types of medical research conducted around the world. There are many other sorts of ancillary-care context we need to consider and many other sorts of questions we need to ask in doing so. These questions are forced on us largely because the contexts of medical research are so varied. An important challenge for the partial-entrustment model of researchers' special ancillary-care obligations— or, indeed, for any model thereof—is whether it can appropriately handle this wide range of contexts. Surely no model will handle all of the contexts perfectly. I will try to indicate as I go through some of these questions, however, where the partial-entrustment model offers helpful resources for dealing with many of them. Some of these questions are conceptual and some are empirical.

Approaching these issues as I have been, the fact that many further conceptual questions open up is a side effect of the broad way that Belsky and I initially defined the problem. We set out to think about medical researchers' ancillary-care obligations, whether these arose in a drug trial for cryptosporidial diarrhea involving HIV sufferers in Zambia; in observational studies of mothers and children with malaria in Tanzania; in "washout" studies of a new antidepressant in Bethesda, Maryland; in studies of new protocols for heroin addicts in inner-city Detroit; in genomic cancer studies in Amsterdam; in brain-scan studies in Boston of moral reasoning; or in multisite trials of palliative-care procedures. Chapter 3's grounding of special ancillary-care obligations in moral entanglements arising from privacy waivers supports this broad approach, for it suggests both that, on the one hand, medical researchers' special ancillary-care obligations are an instance of a (relatively neglected) sort of obligation that crops up in many areas of life and that, on the other hand, this sort of potential obligation is initiated in a quite distinctive way when someone signs up as a human subject of medical research. Hence, addressing the whole sweep of "medical research" is conceptually appropriate. Yet there are important morally relevant differences among the many sorts of research done and the many different contexts in which it is done. Further work on researchers' ancillary-care obligations will need to start to sort out these differences in order to drill down below the level of abstraction at which my presentation has so far been operating.

Here, all I can do is to give a slight foretaste of how this might go, sketching some dimensions of variation that pose challenges to further thinking about ancillary care. The dimensions I will discuss in this chapter are the following:

1. What does it mean to "provide ancillary care" in different parts of the world?
2. Who are the "researchers"?
3. Who are "participants"?
4. What are some of the important boundaries of "medical research"?
5. What if ancillary non-medical problems are encountered?

Important difficulties lurk under each of these headings. I mean to highlight, not minimize, the need for future work along each of these lines. Nonetheless, where I can, I will try to indicate how the partial-entrustment model might help one get a handle on the issues that arise.

Things are otherwise with the empirical questions that need further work. Our collective ignorance about medical researchers' ancillary-care practices and about their attitudes, and about the attitudes of participants and potential participants towards ancillary care, is no artifact of the partial-entrustment model. It is simply a deplorable fact. From my point of view, however, as someone defending a distinctive view about medical researchers' ancillary-care obligations, there is something exquisitely awkward about not even knowing whether asking researchers to conform to the view's standard would be raising the bar for them, in general, or rather lowering it. (My sheer guess, for what it is worth, is that there is a category of well-meaning researchers—malaria researchers well funded by NIH, say—who tend to do whatever they can to provide ancillary care and who would continue to surpass any normative standard that became accepted, but that there are also other medical researchers out there who now provide significantly less ancillary care than the partial-entrustment model calls for.) As the conversation progresses about the standards of ancillary care to which researchers should conform, it is imperative that we learn more about what they are already doing. By the same token, we need to get a sense of whether they and others believe that they are not doing enough or, perhaps, are already doing more than they need. Tackling such empirical questions is beyond my own expertise. In this chapter, I will confine myself to a brief reporting of some initial work that has been done or is under way and some brief suggestions about the kind of data gathering that would be particularly useful.

# NEEDED CONCEPTUAL WORK

I will take up the additional conceptual work called for by variation in medical research by pursuing the five questions just set out.

## *What Does It Mean To Provide Ancillary Care?*

The first point on which further work is needed in order to get past the level of abstraction at which the model has been presented so far is the question of what counts as "providing ancillary care." The case of Malaria Researchers and Schistosomiasis, with which I began, invites us to imagine a group of physicians and other staff in an isolated rural area of Africa with no other medical professionals in the vicinity. Even in rural Africa, this picture is somewhat of an oversimplification. There will be some government-run clinics in provincial towns and often a district hospital to which people might turn for treatment. Waits might be long and the number of physicians woefully inadequate to handle the numbers of patients; but, the point is, even in rural Africa this picture of researchers in the bush glides over some complexities as to who might provide needed ancillary care and how the provision of that care might be arranged. I have mentioned a peculiarity of research funded by NIH that stems from the Inspector General's ban on providing care that is "not study-related," namely that well-meaning research teams often instead use the funds to build clinics in which others can provide care. Where there are already clinics not far away, this approach would hardly be optimal; a less constrained collaboration with local authorities and local caregivers would be better.

What is already a bit of an oversimplification in rural Africa becomes a blatant one in places with more medical infrastructure and better access to health care. Ask ancillary-care questions in a tertiary-care hospital in any industrialized nation, and the natural

response will be: "Why is it not sufficient just to refer the participant to the relevant specialist?" Now, one reason for also offering
the Brain Scans case at the outset was to give an example of why
this response might not be sufficient—in that case because of the
danger of false positives arising from non-diagnostic scans being
read by non-diagnosticians. Suppose, however, that we consider
a Phase I trial of a new cancer drug in a country with a generous
system of national health insurance. If, in that context, the blood
work that is done on the drug reveals some potentially worrisome
abnormality of kidney functioning, it probably *will* suffice to refer
the participant to the nephrologist in the research hospital where
the trial is being conducted. In such a context, the special ancillary-
care obligation will tend to shrink down to what is also covered by
the general duty to warn. In some industrialized countries, however—the United States being the prime case—a large portion of
the population lacks adequate health insurance. For instance, in the
Women's Intra-Agency HIV Study, an ongoing observational, longitudinal study conducted in the United States, 11% of the enrolled,
HIV-positive participants were uninsured (Lillie-Blanton et al.,
2010, 1495). Another sort of situation in which U.S. participants, at
least, might well not be covered by insurance for an ancillary-care
need is illustrated by an observational study, undertaken as prepa-
ration for a broader study on lupus, to determine the prevalence of
periodontal disease in those with lupus (some connection being
suspected between the two). It would not be uncommon for people
in the United States to lack insurance for the treatment of the periodontal disease discovered in such a study; yet ancillary care for it
is centrally within the scope of entrustment. Looking beyond the
United States, other countries with otherwise generous national
health insurance are less generous towards guest workers and other
immigrants, who might reasonably be the focus of certain sorts of
medical research. And some populations who could theoretically

draw on national health insurance may need some extra counseling
or outreach to help get them to the care they need. Think, for example, of a study of a new rehabilitation protocol for heroin addicts in
Zurich.

Another sort of ancillary-care effort that may be required of
some medical researchers in industrialized countries is the "return"
of information about an ancillary-care need—say, about a potentially worrisome abnormality or a tentative diagnosis—to study
participants who have given bodily samples that have been stored
in a biobank. Re-identifying and locating these sample donors may
make providing them with the relevant information more difficult
than the simple "heads up!" of a paradigmatic warning.

Where national health insurance systems are generous, waiting times can be long. This obstacle in itself can provide a practical focus for the special ancillary-care obligation. For instance, one
study conducted by psychiatrists in Sweden revealed an acute need
for psychoanalysis in some of the participants. The researchers were
troubled about what to do about this, on account of the fact that
waiting times for psychotherapy in Sweden were quite long.[1] As
I argued in Chapter 6, researchers' ancillary-care obligations can
provide reasons that compete with those of impartial justice, calling for some departure from impartially fair allocations of health
resources. I do not know if this Swedish psychotherapy case is such
an instance, but I am sure that it raises this issue.

Even where specialized medical care is freely available, there can
be many ways in which researchers could at least help by facilitating
ancillary care for their participants. As we attempt to think more
concretely about this, one particularly useful category, I suspect,
will be that of the "assisted referral." In an interview study, Barsdorf
and colleagues have explored the value of assisted referral with staff

1. I am grateful to Wlodek Rabinowicz for this example.

members and patients at rural primary clinics in KwaZulu-Natal, South Africa. They quote one clinic attendee, a 37-year-old man, about the difference such assistance can make: "They [trial participants] can get treatment from the clinics, where they [researchers] would have made arrangements" (Barsdorf et al., 2010, 85). Within a major tertiary-care hospital in an industrialized country, referrals can work quite smoothly. In places where the medical resources are more overburdened and the population is less medically savvy, I imagine, assistance with a referral can surely be crucial. With the referral, the researchers can both convey that the care is in fact needed and provide some detailed medical information that may help with its provision. One research team, which conducts public-health studies in four developing countries, has written of the need to help participants with "negotiations for emergency medical care" (Osrin et al., 2009, 777). To be sure, what sorts of assistance in referral are needed for what kinds of ancillary-care needs and whether the assistance in referral that is offered tends to be as innocently informational as I have described it are themselves issues on which more empirical information is needed. Pending such results, we should simply keep in mind the intermediate category of an assisted referral, as falling in between the research team's actually providing the ancillary care and its simply referring a participant to the appropriate specialist.

## Who Are the Researchers?

Off and on, I have alluded to the fact that most medical studies involving human subjects are carried out by teams of people with varied expertise. Similarly, I have adverted to the distinctions among the investigators, the institutions to which they belong, and the sponsors of the research (which may or not be different from the investigators' employers). One might also think about the roles of the indirect funders of the research—such as national governments—and about the local medical hosts, who may provide expertise, medical resources, and access to potential participants. These local medical hosts might, in turn, variously be a national medical research council, a national or district government, or a hospital or medical school. In initially presenting the partial-entrustment model, Belsky and I knowingly abstracted away from all of these institutional differences and spoke instead of "researchers." In this book, I have largely followed that practice. To move ancillary-care debates farther, however, it will be necessary to drop this abstraction and to start to think more concretely about the responsibilities of different institutional actors.[2]

Complicating this institutional picture still further is the fact that many important studies are conducted simultaneously at many different sites. Multisite trials have become so prevalent that, early in 2010, the U.S. Food and Drug Administration issued draft IRB guidelines in which the new elements largely addressed the issues that they raise (FDA, 2010). Integration and coordination across such a study's different sites raises many novel problems—for example, for studies involving imaging technology, regarding the compatibility and interoperability of the imagining technology in use (Langer & Bartholmai, 2010). We must expect that it will be equally common for the different sites of a single multisite study to encounter quite different ancillary-care issues. This might be because of differences in the diseases and other morbidities that prevail in the various locations. It might be because of differences in the medical infrastructure in the different places. Or it might be because of differences in the health-insurance regimes of the different host nations. Consider a hypothetical trial of a new vaccine for

2. Maria Merritt made a good beginning at such an institutional look at the issues in her presentation at the 2006 Georgetown workshop on the Ancillary-Care Obligations of Medical Researchers Working in Developing Countries.

West Nile virus with sites in Egypt, Uganda, and the United States. The U.S. participants who show up with ancillary-care needs may require only a referral to the appropriate specialist. The Ugandan participants who show up with similar problems may have no source of care aside from whatever the research team provides. The Egyptian participants might find themselves in a position intermediate between these other two.

This kind of disparity raises an interesting challenge for the partial-entrustment model.[3] At the level of the scope requirement, the partial-entrustment model rests matters on a study-by-study factor: What matters is the study protocol, which is presumably basically the same across the different sites. The set of study procedures, as set out in the protocol, determines the scope of researchers' special ancillary-care obligations. In the hypothetical West Nile vaccine study, these procedures will be the same in Uganda, Egypt, and the United States. At the level of the strength test, however, the partial-entrustment model individualizes the considerations to a given person's claim for a particular sort of ancillary care. Hence, the participants in Uganda, being more AC-dependent than those in the United States, will have stronger ancillary-care claims and hence more ancillary-care claims that—according to the model— ought to prevail. This result intuitively seems defensible, but does raise questions as to the fairness in treating differently the ancillary-care claims of participants in a single study. This kind of issue will require more thinking.

More generally, attention to the many institutional layers of most medical research will require us to think through more thoroughly where the special ancillary-care obligations reside. At an abstract level, the partial-entrustment model attributes them to *those who*

3. For an important discussion of challenges posed by multisite or "multi-community" studies to a more rights-oriented approach to ancillary-care issues, see Brownsword (2007).

*obtain privacy waivers from the participants in order to proceed permissibly with the study.* But who—or, perhaps better, what entity—is it who obtains these waivers? One way to think about this question is the way the lawyers would. We know from *Grimes v. the Kennedy Krieger Institute* (2001) that, for some legal purposes, at least, it is the sponsoring institution that is deemed to be carrying out the research (cf. Mastroianni & Kahn, 2002). This (in)famous case involved epidemiological researchers at Johns Hopkins's institute devoted to problems of lead poisoning. They had conducted an experiment in Baltimore in which residents of wholly lead-infested apartments were recruited and were moved in to one of two types of apartment: ones that were entirely free of lead paint and ones from which the lead paint had been removed just from the areas most dangerous to children, such as the window frames. Like HIV-vaccine trials, this experiment did not put anyone at increased medical risk. Yet some of the participant families sued, arguing, among other things, that the researchers had not warned them firmly enough about the seriousness of the elevated lead levels that some of the children showed up with. The university's lawyers infuriated the Maryland appeals court by taking the line that the researchers had no special duty of care towards these participants in their public-health study. Thus infuriated, the court handed down an immoderate decision. I by no means wish to defend the court's decision in all its details. I do want to point out in passing that the university's lawyers would not have made this strategic mistake if they had taken to heart the truths behind the partial-entrustment model. According to this model, researchers do indeed have a special duty of care towards trial participants, a duty that stands independently of whether the researchers have harmed them.

More to the present point, which concerns whose duty this is, is the fact that the defendant in this lawsuit was Johns Hopkins University, not the research team as such. This is unsurprising, as lawyers and their clients follow the money; but it also may suggest something about the appropriateness of asking research sponsors to answer for ancillary-care obligations. As a practical matter, in the first instance, it makes sense to think of the principal investigators as bearing the ancillary-care obligations. It is they who must present the protocol to the REC or IRB for approval. Institutionally backing this up in many cases, however, is likely to be an obligation held by the research sponsor. It would be useful to have some empirical research, in relation to this conceptual matter, reviewing protocols to see who is designated as the permittee in the informed-consent documents. Does the fine print typically say that the participants give the needed permissions to the principal investigators? Or does the fine print designate the institutional research sponsor as the recipient of the privacy waivers, using some such language as the following: "We hereby permit the lead-hazard abatement team of the Kennedy-Krieger Institute, acting as an agent for Johns Hopkins University, to..."?

One issue in which a clearer conceptual understanding of these institutional issues would be particularly helpful would be with regard to the ancillary-care obligations that attach to research on banked samples.[4] Often, fluid, tissue, or genetic samples collected in one study are then banked and used in different studies by the initial investigators or in subsequent studies by wholly different teams of investigators. Most commonly, discussions of ancillary-care obligations in this context arise under the rubric of "incidental findings." An "incidental finding" has been defined as "a finding concerning an individual research participant that has potential health or reproductive importance and is discovered in the course of conducting research but is beyond the aims of the study" (Wolf et al.,

---

4. This passage benefited from discussions with Mildred Cho as we were preparing Richardson and Cho (2012).

2008, 219). Being beyond the aims of the study makes the discovered need ancillary in the general sense set out at the outset of
Chapter 3. If the need is discovered in the course of conducting
research—that is, by carrying out research procedures—then this
need falls within the scope of the special ancillary-care obligation,
according to the partial-entrustment model. In an article, I have
argued that the topic of incidental findings, so understood, largely
overlaps with that of ancillary care (Richardson, 2008a, 259–260).
Building from that initial observation, the article also argues that
there is no moral requirement for researchers to go looking for incidental findings—or, more specifically, that the theory behind the
partial-entrustment model does not support any such requirement.
As I would now put it: The idea of unintended, privacy-based moral
entanglements explains obligations that one falls into when engaging with private information about another; it does not call for one
to delve further into that private information in order to find yet
more undiscovered needs.[5]

The issue of potential ancillary-care issues arising from material
in biobanks seems usually to come up under the heading of incidental findings, rather than the related one of ancillary care. This is for
I think two main reasons. One is that such biobanks are typically
organized in and recruit most of their donors from advanced industrialized countries. As we have seen, the ancillary care that research
participants from such places need often shrinks to a warning and a
referral. The other is that the secondary researchers are often based

---

5. There are, to be sure, many nice conceptual questions about how to draw this line. My
favorite metaphysical question in the whole area of ancillary care concerns what the
difference is between "reading a test that has already been carried out" and "doing a
new test," a difference that seems to many to be morally relevant. Suppose that the test
in question was a virtual colonoscopy. The machine is now storing imaging results of
the whole lower torso. Is reading those images with something other than the colon in
mind "reading a test that has already been carried out" or "doing a new test"? How could
one tell? From the point of view of the partial-entrustment model, what would matter is
whether making such a reading would require asking for a new permission.

somewhere geographically quite distant from the donors. However we label the issue, though, the case of secondary research with banked samples raises interesting and difficult ethical issues. How, exactly, the special ancillary-care obligation is conceptualized will make a difference to what it implies about any such later ancillary-care obligations arising at one remove.

Consider the difference in this regard between the partial-entrustment model and Miller, Mello, and Joffe's approach to the general incidental findings issue. Their approach is similar to that of the partial-entrustment model in many respects, but they stress, as one of three necessary preconditions of any obligation to deal with ancillary-care issues arising from incidental findings, the existence of a professional relationship between the participant and the researchers (Miller, Mello, & Joffe, 2008, 276).[6] Now, they seem not to have had the case of secondary research on banked samples primarily in mind. The trouble is that, in those cases, there is no discernible "professional relationship" between the participants and a subsequent team of researchers that has obtained permission to do research using the banked samples. What there may be, however—and what the partial-entrustment model would focus on—is a chain of permission-giving or rights-waiving that links the participants to the secondary researchers. The participants had to give permissions to the biobank (or to the initial researchers who stocked it) to allow subsequent research to be done with the samples, thereby transferring both some powers and—as the partial-entrustment model emphasizes—some responsibilities to the biobank (whether indirectly or in two steps). At least, such responsibilities would arise where the irrevocability of the samples' anonymization does not definitively

6. For some additional comments about the close relationship between the partial-entrustment model and the view put forward by Miller, Mello, and Joffe, see 35n. and p. 37, above.

rule out recontacting the donors.[7] For the secondary researchers to do work with those samples, they in turn have to gain a permission that is dependent on that first permission having been given. Thus it seems likely that the partial-entrustment model—unlike the approach of Miller, Mello, and Joffe—could explain how the secondary researchers could have ancillary-care obligations (if only of the warn-and-refer kind) to the participants (sample donors). Beskow and Burke (2010) have argued, on the basis of the partial entrustment model, that they do, albeit weak ones. Again, though, this whole set of issues requires further conceptual investigation.

The big question that needs to be thought through, in this connection, is how the transferring of responsibilities carried out by this chain of permission-giving is affected by the revocable anonymization of the samples. On the one hand, the material in the bank was covered by the participant's privacy rights before it was donated. Now, however, that it is sitting anonymously there, it is a question whether any further transfer impinges on those privacy rights. Where there is any question of returning important subsequent results to the donor—which is the question on which those writing about incidental findings from biobanks mainly focus (e.g., Meyer, 2008; Knoppers & Laberge, 2009)—it would seem that perhaps the donors' privacy rights are indeed still at stake, since returning the results would require undoing the anonymization.

---

7. Conversely, if research involves only anonymized samples and if returning results to sample donors is effectively impossible either because the key for deciphering the anonymization has been destroyed or because its decipherment is firmly prohibited, then it may well make sense to say, as the U.S. Office of Human Research Protections has done, that the research no longer involves "human subjects" (cf. Clayton, 2005, 16). For a more detailed attempt to bring the partial-entrustment model to bear on secondary research done with banked samples, see Richardson and Cho (2012).

## Who Are "Participants"?

People who donate tissue, fluid, or genetic samples for medical research purposes are clearly participants in medical research. So, too, are the babies born to the participant women in a study of mother-to-child transmission of, say, HIV or malaria. That the babies were as yet unborn when their mothers gave permission on their behalf does not change this. Someone who simply presents himself or herself at the research clinic, without having enrolled in a study, is not a research participant. Some more difficult cases for drawing this boundary are presented by family members in studies that call for home visits. Public-health researchers, whom I will discuss more fully in the next subsection, often find themselves in homes doing interviews (cf. Merritt, Taylor, & Mullany, 2010). There will often be a primary interviewee, but the rest of the family will often crowd around, some wanting to raise issues of their own. More broadly, medical researchers working on observational or interventional trials can find themselves in someone's home. Arguably, even if the primary participant has a moral right to permit the researchers to enter the home, other family members also find their privacy impinged upon. Consider the following case:

> *The Participant's Feverish Child:* Suppose that, as part of a study of a new palliative protocol for HIV-related wasting being conducted in a district capital of an African country, the researchers visit the participants in their homes rather than requiring them to undertake the trip to the hospital. On one of these visits, while in the participant's one-room hut, the visiting researcher notices that one of the participant's children is bedridden with an apparently high fever—likely, in that area, to be malaria. Does the researcher owe this child any more of a response than she would to any non-participant in a similar condition?

In this case, the child did not sign up for the study—but neither did the babies born during mother-to-child transmission studies. And as with those babies, this child's privacy rights were partially waived on her behalf by a parent. Perhaps we should not get hung up on the term "participant," but instead ask to whom researchers owe special ancillary-care obligations. If Chapter 3's rationale for the partial-entrustment model is on the right track, then the participant's feverish child, it seems, should be included in that group, because its privacy rights have effectively been waived for it by its parent. This kind of question, however, deserves further conceptual investigation.

For now, though, I leave it behind and turn to a broader and practically very significant set of people about whom one might reasonably be in doubt whether to classify as research participants or not, namely those who attempt to sign up to participate in a study but who are determined ineligible for one reason or another. In most clinical trials and some epidemiological ones, potential participants are subject to a careful, protocol-defined process of screening. This screening can range all the way from posing a few questions to doing a complete "work-up" that includes taking a full medical history, running a battery of tests, and conducting a full physical examination. Depending upon what the screening reveals, some of those people screened will end up being accepted into the study. In their cases, the researcher–participant relationship will be fully established, and any obligations that apply within this relationship will come fully into force. Some people, however, will end up being screened out because these questions, tests, or examinations trigger one or more of the study's exclusion criteria. Often, this will be because these procedures reveal that the individual has some other disease or condition that would either confound the study data or pose a safety danger. Alternatively, the screening might reveal that the disease or condition under study has simply become too serious in this individual for him or her to be included in the study.

In relation to both of these groups of people—the screened-out and the enrolled—the screening phase presents a challenge to any account of researchers' ancillary-care obligations that is, like mine, keyed to what the researchers find out by interacting with individuals in the ways that their protocol requires. Because screening work-ups can be so thorough, and are often designed to discover what other potentially worrisome medical conditions an individual may have, they are apt to turn up lots of different ancillary-care needs. In many contexts—though this question, too, needs empirical study—we could surely expect the screening phase to turn up more ancillary-care issues than would the main body of the study. If the special ancillary-care obligation extends to what is discovered during screening, then it is more extensive than one might have thought. If, further, it extends to individuals who are determined ineligible for participation in the main study, that would be a dramatic implication. Here, I will focus on the screened-out, keeping in mind in the background the broader issues about screening.

In the previous chapter, I briefly set out what I take to be the main implications of the partial-entrustment model for the case of those who have been determined ineligible to participate in the main study. We must recognize, to begin with, that needs that are discovered in the course of screening fall within the scope of the special ancillary-care obligation. Taking individuals' medical histories and doing initial screening tests on them requires their permission, waiving their privacy rights, just as do the procedures of the main study. Hence, the basis on which the partial-entrustment model rests researchers' special ancillary-care obligations is definitely present in the case of those screened out. As I suggested in the previous chapter, however, these needs discovered during screening are only minimally within the scope of what these individuals entrust to the researchers. (This conclusion holds equally for those screened out and for those who end up being enrolled.) That is because possible variations in the exclusion criteria are less central to the study's design and purpose than are its endpoints or its principal design features (such as its distinction between intervention and control arms or its planned stratification of its participants). Still, being "minimally" within the scope in this way puts claims that arise from screening information, as far as this goes, on a par with claims arising from conditions fortuitously encountered by carrying out study procedures, such as finding schistosomiasis in participants in a malaria study. Another point about the ancillary-care claims of those screened out is that, according to the partial-entrustment model, they will, other things equal, necessarily be weaker than similar claims by those enrolled. That is because, necessarily, the depth of the relationship between the individual and the researchers, insofar as this is predictable on the basis of the protocol, will be lower in the case of those screened out than it is in the case of those screened and enrolled.[8]

When researchers carry out screening procedures, sometimes they will reach diagnoses of which the screened individual was unaware. Sometimes, however, what they conclude will already be known to the individual. Does it matter to the researchers' responsibilities whether the diagnosis they reach is news to the individual? That it is not news to the individual does not negate the privacy-based rationale of the partial-entrustment model. Revealing to the researchers who have asked about one's medical history that one is HIV positive, or has herpes, or whatever, will be just as effective a way of entrusting the researchers with some duty to care for that

---

8. If a study requires any pre-enrollment screening, it will generally not enroll anyone without screening them.

condition as will be permitting the researchers to test for one's HIV status, or herpes, or whatever.

If the diagnosis that the researchers reach is news to the individual, however, that will automatically deepen the intimacy of the transaction, and hence the depth of the relationship. It will also heighten the potentially autonomy-threatening effects that, I argued in Chapter 5, provide reasons why it is generally wrong to seek anticipatory waiver of ancillary-care claims. Consider again the case of HIV testing. It is widely recognized that, where HIV testing is conducted, counseling should be offered for those who are found to be HIV positive. This recognition reflects not only a strong call for compassion but also a higher level of intimacy than obtains when individuals simply supply the information, already known to them, that they are HIV positive. The latter can be appropriately done impersonally, on a form. Conveying to someone the news that he or she is HIV positive, on the other hand, has to be handled with far greater sensitivity and tact, and brings the messenger and the recipient of the news into a more intimate relationship. The case of HIV is dramatic in this respect, but not exceptional. This greater intimacy is just the sort of factor made central by the partial-entrustment model. Although the model thus tends to imply that there would be an important differentiation between screening results that are news to the individual and those that are not, this matter, too, requires further conceptual investigation.

## What Are Some of the Important Boundaries of "Medical Research"?

The rationale for medical researchers' special ancillary-care obligations developed in Chapter 3 clearly implies that similar ancillary-care obligations arise in all walks of life. At almost any moment, in interacting with other people, we are apt to get entangled in special duties of care that arise out of accepting others' invitations to enter into their private concerns. As I have mentioned, however, the ancillary-care obligations arising in medical research are distinctive in that there is a sharply defined, institutionalized process wherein the relevant privacy waivers are accomplished, namely the informed-consent process. Now that we turn to examining, more closely, the borders of medical research, we must make this point more precise. Strictly speaking, the informed-consent process applies to any research involving human subjects. Here I will examine two types of research involving human subjects that are not ordinarily considered "medical": public-health research and social-science research. In Chapter 2, I deferred such discriminations, suggesting that we broadly understand "medical research" as "any kind of scientific research that enrolls human participants and that concerns itself with the workings of the human body." That broad reading counts as "medical research" a version of Brain Scans in which the investigators are philosophers interested in how the brain functions when grappling with ethical problems. Now, as we explore unsettled questions requiring further conceptual work, it is time to drop this stipulated usage and be more deferential to how the term "medical research" is in fact used.

The field of public health is itself vast and varied and raises a number of distinctive ethical problems of its own.[9] The mission of public-health interventions, like the mission of medical research, is directed towards benefiting a collective—a local community, if not humanity as a whole. Unlike medical research, the subject matter of public-health work is also collective, concerning such matters as the behavior of certain diseases in populations with certain characteristics. This collective focus of public-health work generates

9. This paragraph and the following discussion of the cholera clinic in Sudan draw on Richardson (2010).

some truly difficult ethical quandaries regarding whether and when promoting the public good can justify impositions on individuals' basic liberties, such as forcibly quarantining people with dangerous infectious diseases (cf. Corrado, 1996). Whether to use triage and other priority procedures to sort among individuals in allocating resources in a public-health effort is not one of these difficult quandaries. For instance, when authorities are faced with an incipient flu epidemic, if supplies of flu vaccine or antivirals are limited, it is presumably not only permissible but also morally required for the authorities to ration the supply in some reasonable way. What particular principles should apply to their allocation will be a more controversial question (cf. Persad et al., 2009); but *that* they may be denied to some and offered to others on some basis reasonably related to public health is beyond question.

That public-health work is oriented in this way to the good of the public is thus one of its defining features. Here, I want to explore two different types of public-health work, each in a different way exemplifying this focus on the public. One type, which is addressed to public-health emergencies, is not research at all, but departs from being "clinical," in the ordinary sense, because of this kind of focus on a public problem. Another type is community-based public-health research, in which the "subject" really is the community, more than any individual in it.

Delan Devakumar (2010, 53) has described the predicament of those working in a Doctors Without Borders clinic set up some years ago in Juba, a district capital in then civil-war-wracked southern Sudan, to help combat a cholera outbreak. The doctors were given the following instructions:

> So the plan is, if someone comes in to our Cholera Treatment Center with anything other than cholera, you just transfer them to the hospital nearby. And if they have cholera plus

something else you can keep them…depending on how bad the other thing is, otherwise transfer. The reason being that we are just here for the cholera and don't want to take over the work of the Ministry of Health. Oh yes, and we generally don't provide transport. The hospital has lots of ambulances that they do not use.

Understandably, many of the staff were uncomfortable about this limitation. Very many of those arriving at their tents with cholera did have other serious problems. Many arrived at the tents not with cholera but with other medical problems in need of immediate attention. Many of the doctors and nurses felt that they had come to the country with a specific public-health mission—to stem the cholera epidemic—and worried about taking in patients without cholera, who would be in danger of contracting the disease from those with it. "The counter-argument," as Dr. Devakumar describes it, was

> that we had a duty of care to our patients. Most agreed with this sentiment, but we were splitting hairs as to who we were defining as patients. If they only get to our Admissions tent, were we obliged (both legally and morally) to treat them? Rather than trying to treat a patient holistically, we were confining ourselves to one of their ailments; like doing medicine with blinkers on. "I don't care about your cough, I just want to know how much diarrhea and vomiting you have."

Thus, these doctors and nurses were torn between their public-health mission and the responsibilities they felt towards the specific individuals in front of them.

Now, it is an important conceptual question whether the partial-entrustment model of medical researchers' special ancillary-care obligations is also an appropriate basis for addressing the ancillary-care obligations of such public-health professionals who are *not* engaged in research. Perhaps because of my own philosophical bent, I am most impressed by the abstract similarities of the two contexts. To begin with, in this kind of public-health work, the public purpose of stemming an epidemic stands in for the researcher's purpose of contributing to general knowledge. Each of these laudable aims is directed towards the public's good and each provides a good reason to resist assimilating the duties of the relevant professionals to those of a primary-care physician or other clinician. In addition, both medical researchers and these public-health professionals are engaged in transactions with individuals that require those individuals to cede their privacy rights. Once one of these public-health workers begins examining one of those who have come into the tent, this boundary of privacy has already been crossed. If, in thus examining someone, the public-health professional discovers other problems besides cholera, these are ancillary-care needs: ancillary in relation to the cholera-stemming purpose of the interaction (at least as it is understood on the organizers' side). Arising from an examination that required permission, these ancillary-care needs are within the scope of entrustment. Of course, there are also relevant dissimilarities. For instance, I take it that the moment of entrustment, in such public-health contexts, is not nearly as formalized as it is by the informed-consent process required in medical research. It is also clear that the urgent need to stem the cholera epidemic represents a consideration that might well overwhelm most claims to ancillary care. (In the partial-entrustment model, this consideration would enter under the heading of cost, as part of the test of strength.) How much such differences matter to the moral outcome in such cases is an important question for further study.

Turning now to public-health research, I would like to describe the pioneering work of Merritt, Taylor, and Mullany (2010) on community-based public-health interventional research. The case they use to illustrate their points is the Nepal Newborn Washing Study (NNWS). The study question was the difference it would make to newborns' health for them to be washed soon after birth with chlorhexidine-soaked wipes. This is obviously a procedure that could be carried out by whoever is attending the birth. Since the overwhelming majority of the women in the study population give birth at home, this would likely be a midwife or family member. One of the distinctive features of such public-health research, then, as the authors point out, is that it involves this kind of low-tech, often preventative intervention that can be carried out by lay people and certainly does not require the services of a physician. This study also had two other, interrelated features that, these authors suggest, are typical of community-based research on public-health interventions, namely a very large sample size and a deep embedding in the community. The NNWS was set up with a control arm, half the participants receiving wipes without chlorhexidine. All participating mothers, however, were provided with vitamin A and folic acid supplements, tetanus immunizations if needed, prenatal education, a clean birthing kit, and basic neonatal care. The study team recruited 17,306 mother–infant pairs over a thirty-month period. To do so, they needed to recruit and train 475 people from the study population in order to carry out the follow-up visits. As often as eleven times in the 28 days following birth, study volunteers would visit the newborns in their homes to weigh them, assess their breathing, and the like. These study workers, lacking medical training, would not have had specialized competence to diagnose or deal with medical problems; but, spending this much time in the participants' homes, they would have been in a position to notice if someone in the family were ill.

In addressing the ancillary-care questions arising from such a case, Merritt, Taylor, and Mullany focus in part on the basic aids to a safe and hygienic birth that were provided to all participants. These, I would have thought, might well be called for, instead, under the heading of trial safety. They are part of the basic "standard of care" that, from the point of view of the researchers and in light of local resource constraints, should be provided to all participants in order to ensure an adequate standard of safety to all participants. More truly ancillary would be some other condition noticed by one of the home visitors: some problem with the newborn or some illness in someone else in the household. Given the amount of time that the study workers spent in people's homes in this study, it certainly exemplifies the point—made abstractly in the previous subsection—that studies that take investigators into the home can end up impinging on the privacy of others besides those who are officially enrolled in a study. Thus, the embedding of such a study in the community, which Merritt, Taylor, and Mullany emphasize, serves in part to efface the moral importance of the line between official participants and their family members. Allowing this functional impingement on privacy to broaden the scope of special ancillary-care obligations potentially arising from such a study (according to the partial-entrustment model) would allow it to recognize these family members as having special ancillary-care claims on these researchers.[10] Because the vast majority of this study's workers lacked medical training, however, their ability to address any serious medical needs was sharply limited. The authors comment that, "[a]s is the case for most [community-based public-health intervention] studies, it was *ex hypothesi* not feasible for NNWS to muster local physicians, nurses, or other highly

10. Instead of drawing on the partial-entrustment model, Merritt, Taylor, and Mullany emphasize how far one can get, in a context such as that of the NNWS, with the general duty of rescue. I have no quarrel with that effort, and seek here, as in general, to explore the ways in which the special ancillary-care obligation might supplement what the general duty of rescue requires of us.

skilled personnel to provide advanced newborn care to the entire study population." That is to say, the cost of doing so in this case would have been prohibitive: Huge salaries would have to have been offered to recruit such personnel from elsewhere, train them in the local language, etc. (whether such difficulties are typical of public-health intervention studies is another matter on which data are needed). In part because such a case represents such a contrast, if not imbalance, between the scope of potential ancillary-care obligations and their likely strength, this kind of case deserves further conceptual investigation.

Public-health research that is still farther removed from the sort of medical research mainly discussed in this book includes epidemiological research that does not enroll individual subjects but works instead from statistics in the public record. One well-known example of such research is the attempt to identify so-called "cancer clusters" and then, by further examination of the statistical and environmental evidence, to try to determine whether there are specific toxins that might be blamed for the local concentrations of cancers that have been reported. Since such work is based on disease reports that are both anonymized and required by law, they do not require anyone to waive privacy rights. For that reason, the partial-entrustment model of ancillary-care obligations does not apply to them. If such epidemiological researchers have any reason to provide warnings or, say, assisted referrals to any of those living in the designated localities of concern, this would have to be on some other moral basis. If the anonymization of the data is revocable, then the general duty of rescue might apply.

## What if Ancillary Non-medical Problems Are Encountered?

In the case of the NNWS, we have just encountered the crucial difference that the training of the research team members makes to the ancillary-care obligations it is reasonable to attribute to them. This lesson is not, strictly speaking, an application of the general principle that "ought" implies "can," for the sponsors of a study like this *could* have decided to cut their study sample in half (or to forego another study they were contemplating) in order to hire another physician or two. It is rather, as I have suggested, that the cost to the research enterprise of so doing is more than reasonably could have been required of them. Now, in almost all of the examples of medical researchers' ancillary-care duties in this book, there has been a match between the general expertise of the team and the ancillary-care needs they discover (Brain Scans is an exception). In some of the cases, this match is tighter than others. In Malaria Researchers and Schistosomiasis, specialists in one infectious parasite discover another. In the case of the woman in the Rakai community study of STDs and HIV transmission who was discovered with advanced cervical cancer, it was at least within the team's competence to diagnose the problem, even if they lacked the surgical skills and equipment to treat it. In all of these cases, however, the discovered ancillary problem has been a medical one. Yet medical researchers might well discover non-medical problems by carrying out study procedures.

Two such problems are at least suggested by cases that have already been mentioned. One non-medical problem that some medical researchers often come across is that of spousal abuse. In the Welts case, mentioned in Chapter 3, evidence of physical abuse is noticed by a sexual partner. Such evidence might equally be noticed by a researcher conducting a physical exam. Interviews conducted in HIV-transmission studies in order to collect demographic information and information about the participants' sexual practices also commonly elicit verbal reports of sexual and spousal abuse. Because such an HIV study might well employ social workers, either to conduct the interviews or to provide counseling to those found to be

HIV positive, it might well be within the professional competence of this team to provide trained follow-up on such reports. At the very least, they might consider their special ancillary-care obligation to provide these participants with assisted referrals to any local social-service providers that may exist. Another type of research in which medical researchers are very likely to encounter non-medical problems is research enrolling alcoholics or drug addicts. These research participants are apt to have a host of social and economic problems. In addition, these problems are apt to come to light through the research, since these researchers tend to be interested in behavioral and socioeconomic factors that affect the ways their participants cope with their addiction or their rehabilitation.

These are examples of non-medical ancillary care that a medical research team may well be able to provide. Especially where a range of non-medical ancillary-care needs are predictable, however, there may sometimes be a case for hiring some personnel who would be able to cope with them. While doing this falls generally under the rubric of planning for ancillary-care needs—the need for which the following chapter will stress—it is also a possibility that calls for further conceptual investigation, since it highlights the degree to which the partial-entrustment model of researchers' special ancillary-care obligations constructs these obligations directly on a moral basis rather than working within the ethical self-understandings of a given profession. Any call for additional hiring would be a controversial stance. This is another issue that needs to be further debated.

## NEEDED EMPIRICAL WORK

Along the way, while mentioning ancillary-care topics that call for considerable further conceptual work, I have mentioned examples of the need for further empirical study to support that work. These examples indicate the wide variety of empirical work that will be needed to support progress in working out reasonable responses to the challenge of ancillary care. At the most basic level, we need to know about the ancillary-care needs that medical researchers encounter; for example, what sorts of ancillary-care needs show up in the screening phase of studies, and with what frequency? Other empirical questions bear more directly on the conceptual approaches we take to ancillary-care issues, such as the question about whom informed-consent documents tend to designate as the recipient of the participants' rights waivers, the principal investigators or their employing institution. And some bear on the kinds of responses to ancillary-care needs that are being made, might usefully be made, or could be made. One such question is in what circumstances assisted referrals are made and are found useful. Another is how commonly true it is that in community-based public-health intervention studies it would be prohibitively expensive to hire nurses or doctors to cope with the ancillary-care needs that the study predictably will turn up.

Our need for more empirical work related to ancillary care is pervasive. We know almost nothing about what ancillary-care needs medical researchers encounter, how they deal with them, and what they and their study participants think about how they should be dealt with. Fortunately, now, research is being done to begin to collect such data. I have already referred to the attitudinal survey done in KwaZulu-Natal by Barsdorf et al. (2010). These investigators conducted open-ended interviews with 29 adult employees and visitors (patients) at primary-care clinics in this South African province, plumbing their views about whether researchers conducting HIV-vaccine trials should provide HIV care to those participants who become HIV positive during the trial. As these authors note, the results were generally in tune with the partial-entrustment

model's prescriptions: By and large, the respondents, despite rejecting any basis for such obligations in the research having harmed
the participants in any way, nonetheless held that the researchers
should provide, perhaps not all the HIV care that these participants
needed, but some reasonable amount of HIV care, or at least assisted
referrals. This kind of result is very useful both in indicating what
this group of people finds to be reasonable and in helping research
sponsors predict what would result from community consultations
in KwaZulu-Natal on this issue. More such studies are needed. As
I write, a thorough study of ancillary-care attitudes and behavioral
public-health intervention research occurring in facility-based and
community-based research settings, with global reach, is being conducted by Holly Taylor, Maria Merritt, and colleagues.[11]

As helpful as such attitudinal surveys are, it is hard to imagine much progress towards uniform or clear guidance on medical
researchers' ancillary-care responsibilities—whether such guidance
is merely informal and aspirational or more institutionalized—in
the absence of more comprehensive information about the ancillary-care problems actually encountered and about researchers'
actual responses to them. For drug trials, at least, there is a potential
source of such comprehensive information, namely the mandatory
process for reporting any "adverse events" encountered in a trial.[12]
Encountered ancillary-care needs would count as adverse events of
the kind in question, which is purposely defined in a way that pre-
sumes nothing about the etiology of the reported events. Mining

---

11. Holly A. Taylor, Principal Investigator; Maria Merritt, Luke C. Mullany, and
    Louis Niessen, co-investigators. Ancillary Care in Community-Based Research:
    Deciding What to Do. 1 R01 AI085147-01A1 (Funder: National Institutes of
    Allergy and Infectious Disease, National Institutes of Health). Award period
    5/15/2010–4/30/2014.
12. Stephen DeCherney suggested that this source of information be tapped in his pre-
    sentation to the 2006 Georgetown Workshop on the Ancillary-Care Obligations of
    Medical Researchers.

the existing adverse-events databases for ancillary-care information might be possible. This would be a lot easier, however, if the authorities who control the collection of such adverse-events data could be persuaded to add to the required reporting forms a field or two pertaining to the ancillary nature of the disease or condition encountered and to the nature of any follow-up care or action that may have been taken by the research team.

Short of such an official reform in data-gathering, we might at least hope that the various major sponsors of medical research, such as NIH, the Gates Foundation, and the major pharmaceutical companies, might begin to keep track in a systematic way of the ancillary-care needs that they encounter and how their researchers cope with them. Only once this begins to be done will the medical-research community be in a position to deal responsibly with ancillary-care needs.

# Chapter 8

# Philosophical Implications and Practical Steps

Before drawing any broader lessons for theory and practice, let me review the path we have taken. We began with the fact that both medical researchers and research participants tend to think that researchers owe some ancillary care to their participants. This fact, which Belsky and I picked up anecdotally, is now beginning to be confirmed by systematic attitudinal surveys. Probing these thoughts a little further reveals that many think that this "owing" or obligation is something that holds specially between the researchers and the participants in their studies, giving their research participants a kind of claim on the researchers that is not enjoyed by the participants in others' research studies or by the staff in the café that the researchers frequent. The partial-entrustment model captures these thoughts, also honoring the reasons why many—researchers and participants alike—take there to be significant limits to what can be expected of researchers by way of ancillary care. The model captures these limits both by setting a firm boundary to the scope of the special ancillary-care obligation and by setting out a test of the strength of potential ancillary-care claims. The model thus seems to fit reasonably well with our considered judgments about ancillary care, informally gathered.

The model required philosophical reinforcement, however, in order to withstand pressure from two opposite directions: To defend itself against ancillary-care skeptics, it needed a deeper explanation of how a mutually voluntary transaction between researchers and participants could give rise to this sort of additional obligation, so often unexpected; to defend itself against ancillary-care inflationists, it needed a deeper explanation of why its scope is limited to what researchers discover by acting on the permissions they had to collect in order to proceed permissibly with their study. Chapter 3's account of how ancillary-care obligations arise from privacy-based moral entanglements firms up the view on both sides. Addressing the ancillary-care skeptics, it explains that certain sorts of rights waivers also convey important responsibilities. Addressing those who wonder about the appropriateness of the scope limitation, it explains why these special responsibilities remain focused on the vulnerabilities opened up by these rights waivers. In the context of medical research, this means that the scope of obligation centers on the information gleaned by acting on the participants' waivers of their privacy rights to their bodies and their medical histories.

All of these explanations bear on medical researchers' special obligation to provide ancillary care. General obligations of rescue or justice, however, can also support providing ancillary care. I argued in Chapter 4 that although considerations of justice suffice neither to ground a special ancillary-care obligation nor to generate broadly applicable reasons against providing ancillary care, they do often reinforce reasons to provide ancillary care, especially to the group of participants describable as "AC-dependent." These considerations of justice also support Chapter 5's conclusion that there are important moral constraints on soliciting participants' advance waiver of their ancillary-care claims. In addition, as we saw, because those claims rest on an underlying responsibility that has been transferred to the researchers, they are harder to waive than are many other sorts of claims.

The theoretical basis of the partial-entrustment model being thus bolstered, we turned in Chapter 6 to the more practical question of whether the model could be brought to bear on the knotty complexities and myriad variations of actual research studies. Tackling the difficult issue of ancillary care for HIV-AIDS, this chapter showed that the model could generate sensible recommendations that systematically respond to the many relevant differences among studies. This, however, is but one area of illustration. Because of the tremendous range and variety of medical research and because of the unfathomable depth of our ignorance about researchers' ancillary-care practices, Chapter 7 argued, much more conceptual and empirical work is needed before we can hope to have a full handle on the issue of medical researchers' ancillary-care responsibilities.

As we await the day when we have such work in hand, however, we cannot simply postpone all action on ancillary care. For pressing practical reasons, we must proceed on the basis of our current understanding to address the urgent ancillary-care needs that medical researchers face every day. Accordingly, I close this book with some reflections on some of the broader theoretical lessons that have emerged that might help guide our understanding or focus our debates and with some relatively nitty-gritty practical steps that can be taken immediately.

## PHILOSOPHICAL IMPLICATIONS

If the account developed here is on the right track, it is no accident that the topic of medical researchers' ancillary-care responsibilities has been until recently almost entirely ignored by writers on medical research ethics. That is because none of the recognized principles of medical research ethics well fits the issue. Like beneficence obligations generally, ancillary-care obligations call for positive, helping performances. For that reason, the concentration of the medical research ethics establishment on avoiding the exploitation and abuse of research participants helps explain why the ancillary-care issue has been sidelined. Yet unlike beneficence obligations as these are most commonly understood, researchers' distinctive ancillary-care obligations are obligations that are special, not general, in that they hold specially between researchers and the participants in their studies, as a result of what occurred in the informed-consent transaction between the two.

To verify the relative novelty of the partial-entrustment approach, consider the list of ethical principles for clinical research put forward by Emanuel, Wendler, and Grady (2000)—initially seven, and, with developing countries in mind, later expanded to eight (Emanuel, Wendler, Killen, & Grady, 2004). These principles are the following:

1. Collaborative partnership
2. Social value
3. Scientific validity
4. Fair selection of study participants
5. Favorable risk–benefit ratio
6. Independent review
7. Informed consent
8. Respect for recruited participants and study communities

In important ways, my account relies on many of these principles. I shall shortly be stressing the importance of collaborative partnership (1) in planning for addressing ancillary-care responsibilities. Belsky and I took for granted the importance of the principles demanding that research be of social value (2), be scientifically valid (3), and offer a reasonably favorable risk–benefit ratio to

participants (5). For that reason, in defining "ancillary care" in relation to medical research, we stipulated that any care required in
order to make a study scientifically sound or safe would not count
as ancillary care; we wanted to focus attention on care that was
required for other reasons. In arguing in Chapter 4 that provision
of ancillary care would not generally pose a great danger of unduly
inducing study participation or otherwise exploiting participants,
I leant on a division of moral labor with the favorable risk–benefit
ratio (5) and independent review (6) principles. If these two other
principles are adequately attended to, I argued, then providing
ancillary care should generally not pose moral problems of these
kinds. Hence, in these various ways, my account relies on many of
these eight principles. Yet my account of the *basis* of researchers'
special ancillary-care obligations does not lean on any of these principles, nor can any of these principles serve as such a basis.[1]

With reference to their initial list of principles, Emanuel,
Wendler, and Grady (2000, 2708) asserted that:

> these requirements should be sufficient to ensure that the vast
> majority of clinical research is ethical. While it may be impossible
> to exclude the possibility that additional requirements are needed
> in rare cases, these 7 requirements are the essential ones.

In support of this sufficiency claim, these authors cited a leading
text in medical research ethics, which also lacks any adequate basis

---

1. I once thought that the idea of respect for participants as ends, or as "whole persons"—a
specification of principle (8)—might do some important work in grounding their ancillary-care claims. There was a little language to this effect in Richardson & Belsky (2004)
and a broader exploration of this kind of argument in Richardson (2008a, 263). In trying to work this argument out satisfactorily for the present book, however, I encountered
familiar sorts of difficulty in concretizing the Kantian connection between respect for
persons and the idea of treating them as ends. Finding myself unable to surmount these
difficulties, I have here instead rested ancillary-care obligations on the idea of moral
entanglements.

for accounting for researchers' special ancillary-care obligations (Levine, 1986). If the account defended in this book is correct, however, then this claim about the sufficiency of these principles (even as filled out with the one pertaining to collaborative partnership) is not correct. We must add an additional principle, to the effect that researchers must meet their ancillary-care obligations. It is no great criticism of Emanuel, Wendler, and Grady that this ancillary-care principle was left out—especially since as individuals they were as responsible for anyone for bringing issues about ancillary care to the fore.[2] I mention it, however, in order to highlight the fact that practical neglect of the issue of ancillary care seems to have been accompanied by a widely shared theoretical blind spot.

A similar conclusion emerges at a more fine-grained level if we attempt to relate the account developed here to the four well-known principles of biomedical ethics in general (not medical research ethics more specifically) that have been set out and refined by Beauchamp and Childress (2009). Their four principles—which, they stress, need to be differentiated and specified in various ways—are respect for autonomy, non-maleficence, beneficence, and justice. Non-maleficence is not particularly relevant to ancillary care. Justice, by contrast, is importantly relevant but (as I argued in Chapter 4) is not itself a basis for the special ancillary-care obligation. The moral-entanglement rationale for the partial-entrustment model that I have defended here (in Chapter 3) does emphasize the importance and fragility of our capacity for autonomy. In my argument, however, it is the *value* of autonomy and the function of privacy rights in shielding it that do the work. The argument does not hinge on any moral requirement of respect for autonomy or even any moral requirement positively to foster autonomous

2. See the Preface.

decision-making. Instead, the argument conceptualizes special ancillary-care obligations as special obligations of beneficence.

Under the heading of beneficence, Beauchamp and Childress emphasize the importance both of the more commonly recognized obligations of general beneficence and of those of special beneficence. To this extent, the account provided here does fit within their framework. The special obligations of beneficence that they discuss fall into two categories: (1) obligations—often called "associative" (e.g., Dworkin, 1986, 195–202)—that "usually rest on special moral relations (for example, in families and friendships)" and (2) obligations that rest "on special commitments, such as explicit promises and roles with attendant responsibilities" (Beauchamp & Childress, 2009, 205). It is at this level of resolution that the partial-entrustment model, as elaborated here, departs from or amends the framework provided by Beauchamp and Childress. Moral entanglements rest neither on associative ties, such as one's long history with one's family and one's friends, nor on discrete, intentional undertakings of obligation of the kind that occur when making a contract or entering a profession. Rather, they are the unintended results of discrete moral transactions (acceptances of privacy-right waivers) entered into for other purposes (viz., to obtain participants' informed consent). To be sure, especially given their openness to the further differentiation and specification of the principles that they put forward, Beauchamp and Childress could well welcome this account of special ancillary-care obligations as moral entanglements as a friendly amendment supplementing their view.

The category of moral entanglement is equally novel and intriguing from the point of view of moral philosophy in general.[3] It is not only Beauchamp and Childress who leave them out. From the point of view of moral philosophy, what is perhaps most striking about the

3. This paragraph draws on the opening of Richardson (2012).

account developed here is that it shows that this neglected category is practically very important. Given this showing, the category itself will command some interest. Philosophers are well capable of puzzling about even very familiar moral powers. We have the powers to put ourselves under obligations by promising and to relieve others from certain obligations by consenting. As Seana Shiffrin has pointed out, these are intriguing moral powers, in that they are cases in which "the mere expression of an individual's will to alter her moral status can be effective *in just the way she intends.*" In this respect, they contrast with supercilious insults, which may have been intended to assert some form of superiority but are likely to result only in an "unintended duty to apologize" (Shiffrin, 2008, 481). As mysterious as promising can sometimes seem, both the obligation to keep one's promises and the obligation to make amends for a gratuitous insult or other wrong are quite familiar sources of obligation. Moral entanglements, whereby special obligations *unintendedly* arise in a way that is ancillary to some other moral transaction, are interesting and puzzling, too, but for reasons opposite to those pertaining to promissory obligations. Moral entanglements deserve philosophical attention because of the way they involve special obligations arising *without* their having been voluntarily undertaken.

Positioning medical researchers' special ancillary-care obligations in this way as unintended byproducts of a mutually voluntary undertaking importantly provides a potential way to resist the criticism that this kind of ethical constraint on research is overly paternalistic. The way this understanding holds these charges of paternalism at bay is novel and should be of interest both to philosophers interested in paternalism and to specialists in medical research ethics. Accordingly, I will take some space to sketch the two relevant features of the model.

There are many grounds for complaint about the paternalism embodied in standard principles of research ethics. These have recently been well reviewed by Wertheimer and Miller (2007). These complaints arise from a point of view that, reasonably enough, starts by privileging free choice by individuals. A mutually voluntary transaction between two individuals is, absent some special story, regarded as being morally acceptable. By contrast, in the absence of some special, justifying story, state-sponsored or other centralized interference with mutually voluntary transactions in the name of promoting the well-being of the individuals interfered with is criticized as being unacceptably paternalistic. While ordinary commercial transactions may be justifiably subject to some minimal regulation (such as requiring truth in advertising and prohibiting fraud), they are not burdened with informed-consent requirements or requirements of institutional review. Historically, we know why these additional requirements got attached to medical research; but that does not mean that imposing these requirements as a regulatory matter—as they have been—escapes the charge of paternalism.

Rather than pursuing that question further, I want to step back and explain how the moral-entanglements account may help protect medical researchers' special ancillary-care obligations from this charge of paternalism. There are two points, here. First, as I have just noted, the critics of paternalism privilege mutually voluntary transactions and cast suspicion on any special obligations that lack a voluntary basis (e.g., Simmons, 2005). Special obligations that are simply imposed on researchers by regulation thus come under opprobrium. General moral obligations, by contrast, such as the obligation of non-maleficence (the obligation not to harm others), get a pass: All voluntary transactions, it is conceded, must work within the limits these general moral obligations set. The territory mainly explored in this book, namely that of medical researchers' special ancillary-care obligations, thus raises the suspicions of this anti-paternalist camp, for it does concern special moral obligations,

not general ones. Nonetheless, it views researchers' special ancillary-care obligations as arising from their voluntary actions. To be
sure, they arise unintendedly, as duties of reparation generally do
when someone has voluntarily harmed another.[4] Still, they have a
voluntary root. If it could be argued that moral obligations consequent upon actions one has voluntarily taken are no impingement
on one's liberty, then this would already rebuff the paternalists'
criticism. Taking this position would broaden their category of
voluntarily undertaken obligations, but not radically so.

The second point to make in response to worries about paternalism is that, given how the rationale for these privacy-based moral
entanglements refers to the value of autonomy, it should be possible to argue that enforcing medical researchers' special ancillary-
care obligations would fall under the category of so-called "soft"
paternalism, which many critics of paternalism concede to be non-
objectionable (Feinberg, 1971; Feinberg, 1986).[5] That enforcing
these obligations would qualify as soft paternalism is not simply
obvious. Consider how Beauchamp and Childress (2009, 209–210)
characterize the notion of weak or soft paternalism:

> In soft paternalism, an agent intervenes in the life of another
> person on grounds of beneficence or nonmaleficence with
> the goal of preventing substantially *nonvoluntary* conduct.
> Substantially nonvoluntary actions include cases such as poorly
> informed consent or refusal, severe depression that precludes

4. It is *conceivable* that someone might harm others in order to come under an obligation to
provide reparations to them—say, as a desperate attempt to forge *some* sort of relationship with them.
5. In treating "soft" paternalism as basically the same as the "weak" paternalism that
Feinberg introduced in the cited works, I follow Beauchamp & Childress (2009,
235n22). In doing so, I am glossing over the kind of distinction between the two set out
in Dworkin (2010).

rational deliberation, and addiction that prevents free choice and action.

So interpreted, soft paternalism seems to suppose that the person interfered with is, in fact, already compromised.[6] If soft paternalism is interpreted this narrowly, then enforcing special ancillary-care obligations will not fall under it, as the participants' abilities are not yet compromised at the point in time at which ancillary-care guidelines might interfere with their waiving of their ancillary-care claims. Other philosophers, however, have given a somewhat broader reading of soft paternalism while nonetheless continuing to maintain that it is unobjectionable. The relevant broadening is to drop the implication that the person's autonomy must already be compromised and to refer, instead, to what the person would choose if his or her autonomy were not compromised (e.g., Dworkin, 1972; Kuflik, 2010). An example of this approach is Donald VanDeVeer's principle of hypothetical individualized consent. According to this principle, interference with an individual's choices can be justified so long as he would consent if he were fully informed of the relevant facts and his "normal capacities for deliberation and choice were not substantially impaired" (VanDeVeer, 1986, 77). Because this formulation can cover future choices, it is arguably sensitive to the potential threats to individuals' autonomy that might arise after their normal privacy protections have been waived. This is important in relation to my account of special ancillary-care obligations as privacy-based moral entanglements. In explaining the moral basis of those, I have stressed the difficulties a study participant would likely later have if suddenly faced with an unexpected diagnosis.

---

6. I do not claim that Beauchamp and Childress intend this implication. They had spelled it out in the fifth edition of their book (Beauchamp & Childress, 2001, 181), but chose to remove the relevant statement from the sixth.

This is not the place to pursue either of these two points about the potential paternalism objection in any detail. Here, my message is just that the category of moral entanglements intriguingly offers the possibility of resisting the anti-paternalist's critique by resting medical researchers' special ancillary-care obligations in voluntary transactions and by presenting them in such a way that they arguably fall within the rubric of the non-objectionable, soft variety of paternalism.

By positioning medical researchers' special ancillary-care obligations neither as reflecting commitments nor as reflecting associative obligations, I have resisted drawing on a conception of researchers' "professional ethics" in any standard way. This stance, on my part, stems in part from reflecting on the unstable dialectic that Belsky and I encountered when first working on this topic. As I described this in Chapters 1 and 2, this involved a seesawing of responses that either viewed medical researchers, in a peculiarly cramped way, as "mere scientists," or else viewed them, in a quite conventional but inaccurate way, as being akin to personal physicians. In relation to some ethical issues arising in medical research involving human subjects, the profession is indeed well-enough understood: Its ethics has, after all, been regulated for decades. The ancillary-care issue, however, reveals an important wobbliness in the foundations of this understanding. For that reason, it seemed better to construct the argument for researchers' ancillary-care obligations from the ground up, as it were.[7] As it turns out, it has proven practically impossible to abstract entirely from normative understandings of the role obligations of medical researchers. In

---

7. Please do not take this talk of "foundations" and the "ground" as indicating any commitment to justificatory foundationalism, which in fact I reject. In speaking of a profession's "foundation," I take it that I am a long way from the most abstract and general moral principles; and even these, I would argue, must not be thought of as justificatorily foundational. In constructing moral justifications, as Rawls argued (1999b, 18; cf. 19, 507), we are free to prune and adjust considered judgments at any level of generality.

just now cataloguing which of Emanuel, Wendler, and Grady's eight principles my development of the partial-entrustment model takes on board, I noted just how this was so. Yet on the centrally crucial question of what grounds medical researchers' special ancillary-care obligations, my argument avoids presuming any distinctive normative conception of medical researchers' professional role. Instead, the argument hinges on a descriptive observation about what medical researchers must do to get their job done in a way that complies with moral requirements that non-controversially apply to them: They must get permission from the prospective participants to touch them, collect bodily samples, and collect information about their medical histories. This observation does presuppose the normative importance of our privacy rights, but nothing about norms specific to medical research. Hence, instead of centrally relying on a normative understanding of medical researchers' role obligations as a *premise*, my argument seeks to generate some illumination about how those role obligations ought to be understood. Although it was never our ambition in my initial articles with Belsky—or mine here—to provide a comprehensive account of medical researchers' role obligations, I do hope that the account here helps shore up some places where our understanding thereof is weak.[8]

---

8. David Resnik is one who seems to have found some illumination of this kind in my articles with Belsky. He writes (Resnik, 2009) that "Richardson and Belsky's analysis of the investigator-subject relationship is insightful, sophisticated, and well-reasoned. In my judgment, it is the best model of the investigator-subject relationship proposed thus far." While, as I say, it was not intended as offering an overall model thereof, it is nice to think that our account may help people think about this relationship.

Of course, Resnick offers this nicely flattering statement as a prelude to some interesting criticisms. He complains that our appeal to an analogy to bailment is not fully apt, notes the danger that transactionally based ancillary-care obligations might be waivable, and suggests that our account did not pay adequate attention to the limits on the needs a research team is competently able to address. These three concerns have, I hope, been adequately addressed in the current presentation. As I noted at 39n., here the analogy to bailment has been superseded by Chapter 3's appeal to the idea of moral entanglement. As Chapter 5 argues, the concern with waivability is well taken—as these claims are, in

## PRACTICAL STEPS

Even in the absence of a fully worked-out or agreed understanding of medical researchers' ancillary-care obligations, we can agree on important practical steps that need to be taken now to help medical researchers cope responsibly with the issue and to help research participants get the ancillary care they surely should. Because of the neglect that the issue has faced, putting in place even some of the most rudimentary substantive commitments and procedural steps will help immensely.

My confidence in this possibility of interim agreement has some basis in experience. In 2006, we held at Georgetown a workshop on the Ancillary-Care Obligations of Medical Researchers Working in Developing Countries. All but one of the workshop's presenters, joined by a staff member of the AIDS Clinical Trial Group who had been outspoken at the meetings, collaborated to produce a consensus paper, which was published in *PLoS Medicine* (Participants, 2008). This group of authors was highly diverse. In addition to the patient advocate, it included five bioethicists, a law professor, two officials with national research-sponsoring bodies (the NIH in the United States and the Indian Council for Medical Research), three medical researchers (from the United States, Malawi, and Ethiopia), two executives from major pharmaceutical companies, and an executive from the world's biggest contract research organization, which organizes clinical studies for the drug companies.[9]

---

principle, waivable—but not serious, on account of the moral limitations on the waiver of these claims. Finally, as comes out in Chapter 6's discussion of cost and Chapter 7's discussion of the complex institutions within which most medical research is carried out, there are reasons to prefer taking up issues of "ability" via the strength test's scalar dimension of cost rather than as if there were fixed, categorical facts about what a research team is "able" to do.

9. The co-authors and their affiliations were: Roger Brownsword, King's College, London; Allegra Cermak, AIDS Clinical Trials Group, Washington, D. C.; Richard Chaisson, Johns Hopkins University; Michael D. Clayman, Flexion Therapeutics, Inc.; formerly

The practical steps that I will recommend here are all drawn from this consensus paper. Although both this workshop and the resulting paper were focused on ancillary-care needs as they arise most urgently in developing countries, all of the recommendations seem also apt, if possibly less pressing, for the rest of the world.

Before I turn to the practical steps, I would like to describe the principled consensus that this group reached as its basis for practical recommendation. Although of course I hope that my arguments in the foregoing chapters will have convinced many readers, I am also sure that many are not yet ready to sign on to the partial-entrustment model of medical researchers' ancillary-care obligations. For the purpose of responding practically to this urgent and neglected issue, it would be good to locate some useful practical steps that do not require accepting a controversial ethical position.

The workshop's diverse group easily reached a consensus that medical researchers do have significant ancillary-care obligations: that positive obligations to deal with participants' ancillary-care needs are not nil but are not unlimited either. The arguments against an unlimited ancillary-care obligation were the ones we have seen: the unfair and excessive burden on the research enterprise, the threat of undue inducement, and the undercutting of the

Lilly Research Laboratories, Eli Lilly and Company (retired); Peter B. Corr, Science and Technology, Pfizer, (retired) and Board of Governors, New York Academy of Sciences; Stephen DeCherney, Quintiles Transnational Corporation; Christine Grady, Department of Clinical Bioethics, National Institutes of Health (USA); Elizabeth S. Higgs, Division of Clinical Research, National Institute of Allergy and Infectious Diseases, National Institutes of Health (USA); Nandini K. Kumar, Division of Basic Sciences, Traditional Medicine, and Biomedical Ethics, Indian Council of Medical Research; Reidar Lie, Department of Clinical Bioethics, National Institutes of Health (USA); Maria Merritt, Berman Institute of Bioethics and Department of International Health, Johns Hopkins University; Malcolm Molyneux, Malawi-Liverpool-Wellcome Trust Clinical Research Programme, College of Medicine, Blantyre, Malawi; Beyene Petros, Department of Biology, Addis Ababa University, Ethiopia; Henry S. Richardson, Department of Philosophy, Georgetown University, Washington, D. C.; and Jeremy Sugarman, Berman Institute of Bioethics and Department of Medicine, Johns Hopkins University.

host countries' incentive to improve their own system of health care. In thus rejecting an unlimited or extremely expansive reading of researchers' ancillary-care obligations, the group also rejected the claim that such a reading follows from considerations of justice. Yet those considerations of justice, the group found, are among the positive considerations that call for the provision of some ancillary care. Reviewing the group's list of such considerations is an occasion to remind the reader of this book's distinction between researchers' special ancillary-care obligation and other moral considerations that may call for the provision of ancillary care (see Table 1 in Chapter 1). The group did note that "there is considerable consensus that ancillary-care obligations are specially owed to research participants" (Participants, 2008, 3). On this basis, the group was willing to entertain the partial-entrustment model as articulating one possible positive ground of ancillary-care obligation. The three other grounds that the group listed, however, involved general obligations. These were the following (p. 2):

(1) *Due Concern for Welfare*: Due concern for the welfare of those with whom one interacts arguably requires addressing one's research participants' serious medical needs when one has the capacity to do so and they lack other recourse.

(2) *Rescue*: Especially when these needs are urgent, a duty of rescue may come into play.

(3) *Justice*: While it is not up to medical researchers or their sponsors to remedy global injustice in the provision of health care, they do encounter many who suffer from injustices and have some obligation to do their part in alleviating this suffering, where they are competent to do so.

In the foregoing chapters, I have often emphasized the way in which the partial-entrustment account supplements an appeal to rescue, which I tend to see as the operative aspect of due concern for welfare. (The idea of urgency, in the rescue principle, should not be read as implying an emergency requiring quick action; rather, the point is that one can relatively easily help someone and that if one does not, the other person will suffer a significant harm.) And in Chapter 4, I argued that considerations of distributive and rectificatory justice could support or reinforce ancillary care in just the way this group suggests.

Alliterative mnemonics being a prerequisite to punchy and pithy practical proposals, this conclusion that researchers do have positive ancillary-care obligations became the first of this group's "four Ps" of practical advice. These four "guidance points" are the following:

1. **Positive duty:** Researchers and research sponsors, especially those working in developing countries, have some positive moral obligation to provide some ancillary care to their study participants (or to see to it that their participants receive such care).

2. **Planning:** Researchers and research sponsors, especially those working in developing countries, consequently should develop plans, both in general and for each protocol, for meeting the ancillary-care obligations that may be expected to arise. They should also take account of the unpredictable nature of ancillary-care needs and plan accordingly.

3. **Partnership:** These ancillary-care plans should be developed in dialogue and partnership with the host community, in ways that maintain respectful interaction, avoid displacing or disrupting local health-care structures, and represent the population of potential study participants, community advisory boards, and the local medical community.

4. **Practical provisions:** Where they have foreseeable ancillary-care obligations, researchers and research sponsors should take definite practical steps towards meeting these obligations. This might mean hiring a physician with certain competencies as part of the local study team; setting aside a certain line item or percentage of the budget; or forming partnerships with those who can provide drugs or with development agencies that can aid in improving the local infrastructure.

We have seen the principled consensus on which the group rested the first point, which stakes out a rough moral position. Let me now comment on each of the remaining, more purely practical points in turn.

Ancillary-care obligations may be, as I have argued, unintended byproducts of certain moral transactions, but that does not mean that they are either unforeseen or unforeseeable.[10] For example, Libby Higgs, one of the workshop's co-authors, reported the following case (Participants, 2008, 3):[11]

*Mother-to-Child Transmission of HIV in an Observational Study of the Antenatal Effect of Parasitic Diseases:* "[I]n Kenya, a non-interventional study of pregnant women investigated the effect of maternal infection on immunity to various parasitic diseases (such as malaria and schistosomiasis) on their babies. Relying

10. The distinction between what one intends and what one merely foresees as a byproduct of one's action is, of course, at the core of controversies about the doctrine of double effect. Some critics of the doctrine allow that this is a distinction but argue that it lacks the moral significance that the doctrine claims for it (a significance that is not claimed for it by my ancillary-care account). Other critics, however, have cast some doubt on the distinction (e.g., Bennett, 1995, Chapter 11). For an empirically informed reconstruction and defense of the distinction, see Mikhail (2007).

11. I have supplied the case with a name and have fixed a small typographical error.

on published studies of women visiting antenatal clinics in this area, a 30% HIV prevalence rate was expected among study participants. On this basis, it was calculated that administering single-dose nevirapine (then otherwise difficult to obtain) would prevent 11–20 HIV infections among the babies born to study participants."

As this case well exemplifies, medical researchers, who pick their study locations carefully on the basis of demographics and other factors, will generally be quite knowledgeable about diseases and other medical problems that are prevalent where they will be working. Having done so, they will know to expect a certain range of ancillary-care needs. The Ethics Working Group of the HIV Prevention Trials Network has recommended that "systematic assessments be conducted to reveal some of the prevalent health conditions in the local population in order for investigators to anticipate at least some of the ancillary-care needs of study participants" (Rennie, Sugarman, & HPTN Ethics Working Group, 2009, 37). This seems like a good idea for a wide range of studies. In addition, since they will have expert knowledge of their study procedures, they will know what sorts of ancillary-care needs those procedures are likely to turn up. Of course, it might very well turn out that they also encounter some truly rare or unusual disease or condition calling for ancillary care. While researchers of course cannot hire personnel or stock in drugs and equipment to deal with every sort of ancillary-care need that they might encounter, they will nonetheless be able to plan, in a more general way, how to respond flexibly to unforeseeable problems. In remote areas, this can mean being sure to have with them a stock of the medicines deemed by the WHO to be essential in any basic clinic. In an area with a competent but overburdened local hospital, this can mean being sure to have in place a mechanism for assisted referrals.

In a tertiary-care center, this can simply mean hiring a clerical worker to handle referral paperwork.

As we have seen, partnership or collaboration with host communities has been singled out by Emanuel, Wendler, and Grady as a principle of special importance for medical research in developing countries. In part, such collaboration is an additional check against exploiting the people of those countries for the benefit of patients in the developing world. All arrangements need to be public and open. Collaborative discussion of a study's details is a good way to ensure this. In addition, such collaboration provides a way to help redress the imbalance of power that is apt to exist between the host community and the international sponsors of research, thereby making sure that the voices of the host community's leaders and people are adequately heard. And at a more basic, practical level, appropriate partnership can help tremendously with planning how to deal well with ancillary-care needs. Forming appropriate partnerships with the host country's ministry of health, with its hospitals and doctors, and with its local authorities is essential to determining which ancillary-care needs are best met by the research team and which may fairly and appropriately be dealt with by referrals to local clinics or hospitals. Consider the knowledge that Doctors Without Borders already had, going in, about the capacities of the local hospital in Juba, Sudan. Although the first two rationales for partnership—the avoidance of exploitation and domination—are considerably less relevant to medical research conducted outside of developing countries, this last, practical benefit is relevant everywhere. If you are planning a study enrolling heroin addicts in Zurich or in Baltimore, for example, you would do well to forge partnerships with local clinics and local health authorities in order to plan well how to deal with any ancillary-care needs you may encounter in your participants.

The workshop group's list of practical provisions that can be made in advance also has somewhat of a developing-country tilt, but likewise can be adapted for more general application. The basic point is that, since researchers will often be in a position to know that they will face significant ancillary-care needs in their participants, it is incumbent on them not only to acknowledge this in the abstract but also to take practical steps to enable themselves to fulfill their ancillary-care obligations. Now, there is a whiff of paradox, here. According to the partial-entrustment model's test of strength, the easier it is for a research team to deal with ancillary-care needs, the stronger are the participants' ancillary-care claims. One might worry here about a snowballing effect, fearing that the more a research team did to prepare itself for meeting ancillary-care needs, the more it would be obliged to address those needs, and so the more it would be obligated to prepare itself for meeting them, and so on ad infinitum, or until all available research resources were absorbed into the project of providing ancillary care. My response to this worry is that, having now come to the level of practical advice, we also have reached a point at which it is imperative to get beyond the initial simplifying abstractions of the partial-entrustment model's analysis. As I urged in the previous chapter, we need in any case to start thinking about this issue with due attention to the institutions—hospitals, universities, research sponsors, pharmaceutical companies, and so on—within which and thanks to which medical researchers do their work. A research team's efforts to equip itself to handle ancillary-care needs do not occur in a vacuum, but rather occur against a backdrop of grant budgets, institutional regulations, and competitors for the same pool of research funds. The workshop group's "practical provisions" take this on board, suggesting that the practical steps be taken at the level of budget line items, study personnel, and division of responsibilities with other institutions and organizations. These are matters for reasonable negotiation and compromise, not for the rigorous application of a conceptual algorithm.

Even so, there is considerable danger in leaving too much leeway to existing institutions to work things out as they see fit. While individual medical researchers are often very well-meaning and big-hearted, the institutions for which they work all have a basic institutional incentive to concentrate the resources they spend on the research they are conducting and to minimize what is spent on ancillary care. In addition, institutions tend to be conservative or resistant to change. While our deep ignorance about how researchers currently handle ancillary-care needs makes it difficult to say to what extent current institutional practices would need to change for researchers to meet their ancillary-care obligations, I am sure that some important changes are called for. For these reasons, it is crucial that there be a mechanism for bringing critical attention to bear on ancillary-care issues.

A core feature of the partial-entrustment view leads me to recommend review by IRBs or RECs as the most appropriate mechanism. The research protocol is the bridge, here, between theory and practice. According to the partial-entrustment model, the scope of entrustment is set by the nature of the study, as determinable on the basis of the protocol. Hence, rather than institutionally reviewing individual researchers' actions or research sponsors' broader priorities, it makes sense to concentrate the institutional review of ancillary-care obligations and the plans and provisions for meeting them at the level of the protocol. This would not preclude review and examination of individuals' actions (which might be undertaken by Data Safety Monitoring Boards [DSMBs], at least for drug trials) and of the sponsor's priorities (which could be undertaken by internal reviews and by critical examination in the academic and popular press). The protocol, however, should be central. As it happens, we already have in place an institutionalized mechanism for the review of protocols, the IRB or REC.

IRBs and RECs are quite well suited to taking up a review of a research team's plans for meeting the ancillary-care needs it is likely to face. They are used to dealing with the myriad contextual variations from one study to the next. In doing so, they tend to build up a kind of consistency in judgment by comparing a new protocol to the precedents set by others. This way of proceeding well fits the kind of contextual judgment modeled in Chapter 6. The judgments of gradients of the stringency of different ancillary-care claims for HIV-AIDS illustrated there were comparative judgments of a kind that could only benefit from having available a wider set of comparison cases. IRBs and RECs, by virtue of reviewing all of the research protocols arising in their institution, build up a wide and diverse basis for such comparisons. In addition, since these bodies review protocols before a study is conducted, they are well positioned to insist that adequate advance planning be done for how to meet ancillary-care needs.

One worry about relying on IRBs and RECs to handle the review of researchers' ancillary-care obligations is that they were set up to help protect human subjects. Given that historical focus, they may be insufficiently sensitive to the importance of the general aims of science to give a fair hearing to the broader social reasons why ancillary-care obligations are limited.[12] To be sure, the extent to which this would be so is an empirical question. One might imagine that counter-balancing this historical focus of IRBs and RECs is the fact that most members of these boards and committees are themselves research scientists who identify with the social aims of science and understand them from the inside. In addition, as I have just noted, research-sponsoring institutions will tend to look after the interests of scientific research in the broader process of responding to potential ancillary-care claims. Stepping back a bit, one can see this historical focus of IRBs and RECs on the protection of

---

12. I owe this point to Maria Merritt, who also has concerns, which I do not attempt to address here, about insensitivity to what is owed to communities.

human subjects as being a result of the particular way the regulatory regime has developed. As I have mentioned several times, this development has been unbalanced in that it has failed to develop the concerns of beneficence—the sort of concerns ancillary-care obligations reflect. Accordingly, the deeper answer to this concern may be that IRBs and RECs need to be provided with authoritative guidance on ancillary care that supplements the human-subjects-protection focus of the Common Rule. If such guidance were in place, there would be much less reason to worry about IRBs and RECs being one-sidedly pro-participant in their treatment of ancillary-care issues.

DSMBs might play a complementary role to that of IRBs and RECs by systematically collecting after-the-fact data about ancillary-care needs and how they were addressed. That would dovetail with the suggestion I made in the previous chapter that the adverse-event reporting system be tapped as a source of information about ancillary-care needs. As crucial as information collection is, however, the protocol-based advance review that IRBs and RECs are positioned to make well suits them to be the layer at which to institutionalize primary ethical review of researchers' ancillary-care obligations and how they are to be met. Of course, in addition to their accumulating a sense of precedent for their own internal purposes, we may hope that, given the crying need for more widely shared information about ancillary care, IRBs and RECs would share some of this information more broadly.

The working group's consensus paper offered three questions, or groups of questions, to be asked by any REC or IRB about researchers' ancillary-care responsibilities (Participants, 2008, 3):[13]

---

13. Although the consensus paper presents these questions as pertaining to research in developing countries, they are more broadly relevant than that. I quote only the main questions, not the sub-questions, rewording slightly.

1. *Needs.* What ancillary-care needs, if any, are likely to be encountered in this study?
2. *Alternatives:* Can identified ancillary-care needs be met by the existing local health system?
3. *Obligations:* How strong is the responsibility of researchers and their sponsors to address the ancillary-care needs they identify in this study?

Note that, as with the four P's, taking these three questions to be important does not require buying into the partial-entrustment model, with its distinction of scope and strength. Rather, it rests on the broader level of normative consensus reached by the working group. To be sure, if the partial-entrustment model came to be persuasive, it would be easy to specify the first question so that it was explicitly addressed to the likelihood of ancillary-care needs coming to the researchers' attention by means of their carrying out study procedures.

Under the heading of the question about strength, the workshop group suggested many sub-questions that map easily onto the partial-entrustment model's dimensions of strength. Interestingly, though, two of these sub-questions do not. These are the following (Participants, 2008, 3):

- "Is the research study part of a broader set of studies that these researchers or their sponsors are conducting, or aim to conduct, with this host population?"
- "What is the nature and identity of investigators' and funders' institutions, and to what extent would they be able to support the provision of ancillary care?"

Both of these sub-questions help suggest further detail about why the institutional setting of a research team matters so much.

The workshop group's consensus paper concluded that international guidelines (not "specific rules": Participants, 2008, 4):

> should be developed in tandem with policies and guidance addressed to research sponsors, and...should be international, so as to minimize the danger that a country's stringent ancillary-care standards would cause research studies to locate elsewhere.

Given the pervasiveness and the variability of the ancillary-care needs that medical researchers are apt to encounter in their human subjects, it seems unfair to let the burden of working out a morally adequate response fall on the individual investigators or research teams. Guidelines should be developed so that researchers are neither permitted to ignore their ancillary-care guidelines nor forced to fly by the seat of their pants, improvising anew each time an ancillary-care need arises.

The development of adequate guidelines for medical researchers' approach to ancillary-care issues will have to depend upon a robust theoretical understanding of the issue. Although the workshop group's consensus paper indicates that practical steps can immediately be taken on the basis of a simple understanding of ancillary care with which most reasonable people would agree, an authoritative set of guidelines would need to reflect a somewhat deeper sense of the principled basis of ancillary-care obligations. I hope that the present book has contributed to the development of a deeper shared understanding of this basis, if only by making clear to some readers where the partial-entrustment model goes astray. I have attempted to reveal in this book my deepest thoughts on the issue of ancillary care. My unconvinced readers, having voluntarily entered into these ideas by reading this book and having discovered some problems—anticipated or not—with these ideas, now have a special obligation to me, and a general obligation to the research community, to provide an account of how to fix these problems.

# REFERENCES

Allen, Anita. 1988. *Uneasy Access: Privacy for Women in a Free Society* (Totowa, N.J.: Rowman and Littlefield).

Amadi, Beatrice; Mwiya, Mwiya; Musuku, John; Watuka, Angela; Sianongo, Sandie; Ayoub, Aynan; and Kelly, Paul. 2002. "Effect of Nitazoxanide on Morbidity and Mortality in Zambian Children with Cryptosporidiosis: A Randomized Control Trial," *Lancet* 360: 1375–1380.

Angell, Marcia. 1997. "The Ethics of Clinical Research in the Third World," *New England Journal of Medicine* 337: 847–849.

Appelbaum, P. S.; Roth, L. H.; Lidz, C. W., et al. 1987. "False Hopes and Best Data: Consent to Research and the Therapeutic Misconception," *Hastings Center Report* 17 (2): 20–24.

Aquinas, Thomas. 1981. *Summa Theologica*, trans. Fathers of the English Dominican Province, 5 vols. (Westminster, Md.: Christian Classics).

Arneson, Richard. 1989. "Equality and Equal Opportunity for Welfare," *Philosophical Studies* 56: 77–93.

Arneson, Richard. 2000. "Luck Egalitarianism and Prioritarianism," *Ethics* 110: 339–349.

Ballantyne, Angela. 2008. "'Fair Benefits' Accounts of Exploitation Require a Normative Principle of Fairness: Response to Gbadegesin and Wendler, and Emanuel et al.," *Bioethics* 22:239–244.

Barsdorf, Nicola, et al. 2010. "Access to Treatment in HIV Prevention Trials: Perspectives from a South African Community," *Developing World Bioethics* 10: 78–87.

Beauchamp, Tom L., and Childress, James F. 2001. *Principles of Biomedical Ethics*, 5th ed. (Oxford: Oxford University Press).

Beauchamp, Tom L., and Childress, James F. 2009. *Principles of Biomedical Ethics*, 6th ed. (New York: Oxford University Press).

Belsky, Leah, and Richardson, Henry S. 2004. "Medical Researchers' Ancillary Clinical Care Responsibilities," *British Medical Journal* 328: 1494–1496.

Benatar, Solomon R., and Singer, Peter A. 2000. "A New Look at International Research Ethics," *British Medical Journal* 321: 824–826.

Benatar, Solomon R., and Singer, Peter A. 2010. "Responsibilities in International Research: A New Look Revisited," *Journal of Medical Ethics* 36: 194–197.

Bennett, Jonathan. 1995. *The Act Itself* (Oxford: Oxford University Press).

Bennett, S., and Chanfreau, C. 2005. "Approaches to Rationing Antiretroviral Treatment: Ethical and Equity Implications," *Bulletin of the WHO* 83: 541–547.

Benson, Paul. 1991. "Autonomy and Oppressive Socialization," *Social Theory and Practice* 17: 385–408.

Benson, Paul. 1994. "Agency and Self Worth," *Journal of Philosophy* 91: 650–668.

Beskow, Laura M., and Burke, Wylie. 2010. "Offering Individual Genetic Research Results: Context Matters," *Science Translational Medicine* 2 (38) 38cm20. Accessible via www.sciencetranslationalmedicine.org.

Brahmbhatt, H.; Kigozi, G.; Wabwire-Mangen, F., et al. 2003. "The Effects of Placental Malaria on Mother-to-Child HIV Transmission in Rakai, Uganda," *AIDS* 17: 2539–2541.

Brownsword, Roger. 2007. "The Ancillary-Care Responsibilities of Researchers: Reasonable But Not Great Expectations," *Journal of Law, Medicine, and Ethics* 35: 679–691.

Cash, Richard; Wikler, Daniel; Saxena, Abha; and Capron, Alexander. 2009. *Casebook on Ethical Issues in International Health Research* (Geneva: World Health Organization). Available at http://www.who.int/rpc/publications/ethics_casebook/en/ (accessed 4/1/2012).

Christman, John. 1986. "Autonomy: A Defense of the Split-Level Self," *Southern Journal of Philosophy* 25: 19–35.

Christman, John. 2001. "Autonomy and Personal History," *Canadian Journal of Philosophy* 21: 1–24.

Clayton, Ellen Wright. 2005. "Informed Consent and Biobanks," *Journal of Law, Medicine, and Ethics* 33: 15–21.

Cohen, G. A. 1989. "On the Currency of Egalitarian Justice," *Ethics* 99: 906–944.

Cohen, G. A. 2008. *Rescuing Justice and Equality* (Cambridge, Mass.: Harvard University Press).

Corrado, M. 1996. "Punishment, Quarantine, and Preventive Detention." *Criminal Justice Ethics* 15: 3–13.

Council for International Organizations of Medical Sciences (CIOMS). 2002. International ethical guidelines for biomedical research involving human subjects. Available at http://www.cioms.ch/publications/guidelines/guidelines_nov_2002_blurb.htm (accessed 8/16/2010).

Crisp, Roger. 2003. "Equality, Priority, and Compassion," *Ethics* 113: 745–763.

Crouch, Robert, and Arras, John. 1998. "AZT Trials and Tribulations," *Hastings Center Report* 28(6): 26–34.

Daniels, Norman. 2007. *Just Health: Meeting Health Needs Fairly* (Cambridge, England: Cambridge University Press).

DeCew, Judith Wagner. 1997. *In Pursuit of Privacy: Law, Ethics, and the Rise of Technology* (Ithaca: Cornell University Press).

DeCew, Judith Wagner. 2006. "Privacy," *Stanford Encyclopedia of Philosophy*, ed. Edwin N. Zalta, revised Sept. 2006, introduction; http://plato.stanford.edu/entries/privacy/ (accessed 1/30/2010).

Devakumar, Delan. 2010. "Case Discussion: Cholera and Nothing More," *Public Health Ethics* 3: 53–54, doi: 10.1093/phe/phn036.

Dickert, Neal, et al. 2007. "Ancillary-care Responsibilities in Observational Research: Two Cases, Two Issues," *Lancet* 369: 874–877

Dickert, Neal, and Wendler, David. 2009a. "Ancillary Care Obligations of Medical Researchers," *JAMA* 302(4): 424–428.

Dickert, Neal, and Wendler, David. 2009b. "In Reply," *JAMA* 302(22): 2435–2436.

Dworkin, Gerald. 1972. "Paternalism," *The Monist* 56: 64–84.

Dworkin, Gerald. 2010. "Paternalism," *Stanford Encyclopedia of Philosophy*, ed. Edwin N. Zalta, revised; http://plato.stanford.edu/entries/paternalism/ (accessed 8/20/2010).

Dworkin, Ronald. 1986. *Law's Empire* (Cambridge, Mass.: Harvard University Press).

Emanuel, Ezekiel J. 2004. "Ending Concerns about Undue Inducement," *Journal of Law, Medicine, and Ethics* 32: 100–105.

Emanuel, Ezekiel J., et al. 2004. "Moral Standards for Research in Developing Countries: From 'Reasonable Availability' to 'Fair Benefits,'" *Hastings Center Report* 34: 17–27.

Emanuel, Ezekiel J.; Currie, Yolani E.; and Herman, Allen. 2005. "Undue Inducement in Clinical Research in Developing Countries: Is It a Wrong?" *Lancet* 366: 336–340.

Emanuel, Ezekiel J.; Wendler, David; and Grady, Christine. 2000. "What Makes Clinical Research Ethical?" *JAMA* 283: 2701–2711.

Emanuel, Ezekiel J.; Wendler, David; Killen, Jack; and Grady, Christine. 2004. "What Makes Clinical Research in Developing Countries Ethical?" *Journal of Infectious Diseases* 189: 930–937.

Emanuel, Ezekiel J., and Wertheimer, Alan. 2006. "Who Should Get Influenza Vaccine When Not All Can?" *Science* 312(5775): 854–855.

Feinberg, Joel. 1971. "Legal Paternalism," *Canadian Journal of Philosophy* 1: 105–124.

Feinberg, Joel. 1986. *Harm to Self*, vol. III of *The Moral Limits of the Criminal Law* (New York: Oxford University Press).

Fitzgerald, Daniel W.; Pape, Jean William; Wasserheit, Judith N.; Counts, George W.; and Corey, Lawrence. 2003. "Provision of Treatment in HIV-1 Vaccine Trials in Developing Countries," *Lancet* 362: 993–994.

Food and Drug Administration [FDA] (U.S.A.). 2010. "Guidance for IRBs, Clinical Investigators, and Sponsors IRB Continuing Review after Clinical Investigation Approval: Draft Guidance," January, 2010. Available online at http://www.fda.gov/downloads/RegulatoryInformation/Guidances/UCM197347.pdf (accessed 8/19/2010).

Frankfurt, Harry. 1999. "Equality and Respect," *Social Research* 64: 3–15.

Goodin, Robert E. 1985. *Protecting the Vulnerable: A Reanalysis of Our Social Responsibilities* (Chicago: University of Chicago Press).

*Grimes v Kennedy Krieger Institute.* 2001. 366 Md 29, 782 A2d 807, available at: http://www.courts.state.md.us/opinions/coa/2001/128a00.pdf (accessed 8/19/2010).

Hawkins, Jennifer S. 2006. "Justice and Placebo Controls," *Social Theory and Practice* 32: 467–496.

Herman, Barbara. 2001. "The Scope of Moral Requirement," *Philosophy and Public Affairs* 30: 227–256.

Honneth, Axel. 1995. "Decentered Autonomy," in Honneth, Axel, ed. *Fragmented World of the Social: Essays in Social and Political Philosophy* (Albany: SUNY Press): 261–271.

Hooper, Carwyn. 2010. "Ancillary-Care Duties: The Demands of Justice," *Journal of Medical Ethics* 36: 708–711.

Hyder, Adnan A., and Merritt, Maria W. 2009. "Ancillary Care for Public Health Research in Developing Countries," *JAMA* 302(4): 429–431.

Illes, J.; Kirschen, M. P.; Edwards, E.; Stanford, L. R.; Bandettini, P.; Cho, M. K.; Ford, P. J.; Glover, G. H.; Kulynych, J.; Macklin, R.; Michael, D. B.; and Wolf, S. M. 2006. "Ethics: Incidental Findings in Brain Imaging Research," *Science* 311: 783–784.

Jackson, J. Brooks; Musoke, Philippa; Fleming, Thomas; Guay, Laura A., et al. 2003. "Intrapartum and Neonatal Single-dose Nevirapine Compared with Zidovudine for Prevention of Mother-to-Child Transmission of HIV-1 in Kampala, Uganda: 18-Month Follow-up of the HIVNET 012 Randomised Trial," *Lancet* 362: 859–868.

Katzman, G. L.; Dagher, P.; and Patronas, N. J. 1999. "Incidental Findings on Brain Magnetic Resonance Imaging from 1000 Asymptomatic Volunteers," *JAMA* 282: 36–39.

Knoppers, Bartha Maria, and Laberge, Claude. 2009. "Return of 'Accurate' and 'Actionable' Results: Yes!" *American Journal of Bioethics* 9: 107–109.

Kolodny, Niko. 2010. "Which Relationships Justify Partiality? The Case of Parents and Children," *Philosophy & Public Affairs* 38: 37–75.

Kuflik, Arthur. 2010. "Hypothetical Consent," in *The Ethics of Consent: Theory and Practice*, ed. Franklin Miller and Alan Wertheimer (New York: Oxford University Press): 131–162.

Kukla, Rebecca. 2005. "Conscientious Autonomy: Displacing Decisions in Health Care," *Hastings Center Report* 35(2): 34–44.

Lamont, Julian, and Christi Favor. 2007. "Distributive Justice," in the *Stanford Encyclopedia of Philosophy* (online), Edwin N. Zalta, ed., available at http://plato.stanford.edu/entries/justice-distributive/ (accessed 7/18/2010).

Langer, Steve, and Bartholmai, Brian. 2010. "Imaging Informatics: Challenges in Multisite Imaging Trials," *Journal of Digital Imaging*, online: DOI: 10.1007/s10278-010-9282-9.

Lavery, James V., et al. 2010. "'Relief of Oppression': An Organizing Principle for Researchers' Obligations to Participants in Observational Studies in the Developing World," *BMC Public Health* 10: 384–390.

Levine, Robert J. 1986. *Ethics and Regulation of Clinical Research*, 2nd ed. (New Haven: Yale University Press).

Lillie-Blanton, Marsha, et al. 2010. "Association of Race, Substance Abuse, and Health Insurance Coverage with the Use of Highly Active Antiretroviral Therapy among HIV-Infected Women, 2005," *American Journal of Public Health* 100: 1493–1499.

Lurie, Peter, and Wolfe, Sydney M. 1997. "Unethical Trials of Interventions to Reduce Perinatal Transmission of Human Immunodeficiency Virus in Developing Countries," *New England Journal of Medicine* 337: 853–856.

MacKinnon, Catherine. 1989. *Toward a Feminist Theory of the State* (Cambridge, Mass.: Harvard University Press).

MacQueen, Kathleen M.; Karim, Quarraisha Abdool; and Sugarman, Jeremy. 2003. "Ethics Guidance for HIV Prevention Trials," *BMJ* 327: 340.

MacQueen, Kathleen M.; McLoughlin, Kerry; Alleman, Patty; Burke, Holly McLain; and Mack, Natasha. 2008. "Partnering for Care in HIV Prevention Trials," *Journal of Empirical Research on Human Research Ethics* 3:5–18.

Mastroianni, A., and Kahn, J. 2002. "Risk and Responsibility: Ethics, *Grimes v Kennedy Krieger*, and Public Health Research," *American Journal of Public Health* 92: 1073–1076.

McGough, L. J.; Reynolds, S. J.; Quinn, T. C.; and Zenilman, J.M. 2005. "Which Patients First? Setting Priorities for Antiretroviral Therapy Where Resources are Limited," *American Journal of Public Health* 95(7): 1173–1180.

McIntyre, Alison. 1994. "Guilty Bystanders? On the Legitimacy of Duty to Rescue Statutes," *Philosophy and Public Affairs* 23: 157–191.

McNeil, Donald G. 2009. "For First Time, AIDS Vaccine Shows Some Success," *New York Times*, Sept. 24: A1.

Merritt, Maria. 2005. "Moral Conflict in Clinical Trials," *Ethics* 115: 306–330.

Merritt, Maria. 2011. "Health Researchers' Ancillary Care Obligations in Low-Resource Settings: How Can We Tell What Is Morally Required?" *Kennedy Institute of Ethics Journal* 21(4): 311–347.

Merritt, Maria, and Grady, Christine. 2006. "Rationing Priorities for Antiretroviral Therapy (ART) in Developing Countries: 'Justice as Reciprocity' and Post-Trial Access for ART Trial Participants," *AIDS* 20: 1791–1794.

Merritt, Maria M.; Taylor, Holly; and Mullany, Luke C. 2010. "Ancillary Care in Community-Based Public Health Intervention Research," *American Journal of Public Health* 100: 211–216.

Meyer, Michelle N. 2008. "The Kindness of Strangers: The Donative Contract between Subjects and Researchers and the Non-obligation to Return Individual Results of Genetic Research," *American Journal of Bioethics* 8: 44–46.

Meyers, Diana Tietjens. 2000. "Intersectional Identity and the Authentic Self? Opposites Attract!" in Catriona Mackenzie and Natalie Stoljar, eds., *Relational Autonomy: Feminist Perspectives on Autonomy, Agency, and the Social Self* (New York: Oxford University Press): 151–180.

Mikhail, John. 2007. "Universal Moral Grammar: Theory, Evidence and the Future," *Trends in Cognitive Sciences* 11: 143–152.

Miller, David. 2001. "Distributing Responsibilities," *Journal of Political Philosophy* 9: 453–471.

Miller, Franklin G.; Mello, Michelle M.; and Joffe, Steven. 2008. "Incidental Findings in Human Subjects Research: What Do Investigators Owe Research Participants?" *Journal of Law, Medicine, and Ethics* 36: 271–279.

Miller, Franklin G., and Rosenstein, Donald L. 2003. "The Therapeutic Orientation to Clinical Trials," *New England Journal of Medicine* 348: 1383–1386.

Miller, Franklin G., and Wertheimer, Alan. 2007. "Facing Up to Paternalism in Research Ethics," *Hastings Center Report* 37(3): 24–34.

Moseley, R. 1985. "Excuse Me, But You Have a Melanoma on Your Neck! Unsolicited Medical Opinions," *Journal of Medicine & Philosophy* 10: 163–170.

Murphy, Liam. 2000. *Moral Demands in Nonideal Theory* (Oxford: Oxford University Press).

National Institutes of Health (U.S.A.). 2005. "Guidance for Addressing the Provision of Antiretroviral Treatment for Trial Participants Following their Completion of NIH-Funded HIV Antiretroviral Treatment Trials in Developing Countries," Notice Number: NOT-OD-05-038.

Nozick, Robert. 1974. *Anarchy, State, and Utopia* (New York: Basic Books).

Nuffield Council on Bioethics. 2002. *The Ethics of Research Related to Healthcare in Developing Countries* (London: Nuffield Council).

Nussbaum, Martha C. 2000. *Women and Human Development: The Capabilities Approach* (Cambridge: Cambridge University Press).

Nussbaum, Martha C. 2004. *Hiding from Humanity: Disgust, Shame, and the Law* (Princeton: Princeton University Press).

O'Neill, Onora. 1985. "Between Consenting Adults," *Philosophy & Public Affairs* 14: 252–277.

Osrin, David; Azad, Kishwar; Fernandez, Armida; Manandhar, Dharma S.; Mwansambo, Charles W.; Prasanta, Tripathy; and Costello, Anthony M. 2009. "Ethical Challenges in Cluster Randomized Controlled Trials: Experiences from Public Health Interventions in Africa and Asia," *Bulletin of the World Health Organization* 87: 772–779.

Parfit, Derek. 1997. "Equality and Priority," *Ratio* 10: 202–221.

Participants in the 2006 Georgetown University Workshop on the Ancillary-Care Obligations of Medical Researchers Working in Developing Countries. 2008. "The Ancillary-Care Obligations of Medical Researchers Working in Developing Countries," *PLoS Medicine* 5(5): e90 doi:10.1371/journal.pmed.0050090

Pellegrino, Edmund. 2001. "The Internal Morality of Clinical Medicine: A Paradigm for the Ethics of the Helping and Healing Professions," *Journal of Medicine and Philosophy* 26: 559–579.

Persad, Govind; Wertheimer, Alan; and Emanuel, Ezekiel J. 2009. "Principles for Allocation of Scarce Medical Resources," *Lancet* 373: 423–431.

Philpott, Sean; Slevin, Katherine West; Shapiro, Katherine; and Heise, Lori. 2010. "Impact of Donor-imposed Requirements and Restrictions on Standards of Prevention and Access to Care and Treatment in HIV Prevention Trials," *Public Health Ethics* 3: 220–228.

Pincoffs, Edmund. 1971. "Quandary Ethics," *Mind* 80: 552–571

Pogge, Thomas. 2007. "Severe Poverty as a Human Rights Violation," in T. Pogge, ed., *Freedom from Poverty as a Human Right* (Oxford: Oxford University Press): 11–53.

Powers, Madison, and Faden, Ruth. 2006. *Social Justice: The Moral Foundations of Public Health and Health Policy* (New York: Oxford University Press).

Ratzen, R. M. 1985. "Unsolicited Medical Opinion," *Journal of Medicine & Philosophy* 10: 147–162.

Rawls, John. 1971. "Justice as Reciprocity," originally published in S. Gorovitz, ed., *John Stuart Mill: Utilitarianism, with Critical Essays* (Indianapolis: Bobbs-Merrill, 1971); reprinted in John Rawls, *Collected Papers*, ed. S. Freeman (Cambridge, Mass.: 1999, Harvard University Press): 190–224.

Rawls, John. 1996. *Political Liberalism*, rev. ed. (New York: Columbia University Press).

Rawls, John. 1999a. *The Law of Peoples* (Cambridge, Mass.: Harvard University Press).

Rawls, John. 1999b. *A Theory of Justice*, rev. ed. (Cambridge, Mass.: Harvard University Press).

Rawls, John. 2001. *Justice as Fairness: A Restatement*, ed. Erin Kelly (Cambridge, Mass.: Harvard University Press).

Raz, Joseph. 1972. "Voluntary Obligations and Normative Powers," *Proceedings of the Aristotelian Society* suppl. vol. 46: 79–102.

Rennie, Stuart; Sugarman, Jeremy; and the HPTN Ethics Working Group. 2009. *HIV Prevention Trials Network Ethics Guidance for Research* (HIV Prevention Trials Network). Available at www.hptn.org/web documents/EWG/ HPTNEthicsGuidance020310.pdf (accessed 8/16/2010).

Rerks-Ngarm, S., et al. 2009. "Vaccination with ALVAC and AIDSVAX to Prevent HIV-1 Infection in Thailand," *New England Journal of Medicine* 361: 2209–2220.

Resnik, David B. 2009. "The Clinical Investigator-Subject Relationship: A Contextual Approach," *Philosophy, Ethics, and Humanities in Medicine* 4:16. doi:10.1186/1747-5341-4-16.

Richardson, Henry S. 1999. "Institutionally Divided Moral Responsibility," in *Social Philosophy and Policy* 16: 218–249.

Richardson, Henry S. 2000. "Specifying, Balancing, and Interpreting Bioethical Principles," *Journal of Medicine and Philosophy* 25: 285–307.

Richardson, Henry S. 2007. "Gradations of Ancillary-Care Responsibility for HIV-AIDS in Developing Countries," *American Journal of Public Health* 97: 1956–1961.

Richardson, Henry S. 2008a. "Incidental Findings and Ancillary-Care Obligations," *Journal of Law, Medicine, and Ethics* 36: 256–270.

Richardson, Henry S. 2008b. "Our Call: The Constitutive Importance of the People's Judgment," *Journal of Moral Philosophy* 5: 3–29.

Richardson, Henry S. 2009. "The Investigator-Participant Relationship," *JAMA* 302(22): 2435.

Richardson, Henry S. 2010. "Public Health Doctors' Ancillary-Care Obligations," *Public Health Ethics* 3: 63–67, doi: 10.1093/phe/php025.

Richardson, Henry S. 2011. "Interpreting Rawls: An Essay on Audard, Freeman, and Pogge," *Journal of Ethics* 15: 227–251.

Richardson, Henry S. 2012. "Moral Entanglements: Intimacies and Ancillary Duties of Care," *Journal of Moral Philosophy* 9: 376–409.

Richardson, Henry S. Forthcoming. "Revising Moral Norms: A Challenge for Peircean Pragmatism and Other Ideal-Endpoint Views," in *Constructivism in Ethics*, ed. Carla Bagnoli (Cambridge, England: Cambridge University Press).

Richardson, Henry S., and Belsky, Leah. 2004. "The Ancillary-Care Responsibilities of Medical Researchers: An Ethical Framework for Thinking about the Clinical Care that Researchers Owe Their Subjects," *Hastings Center Report* 34 (Jan.–Feb.): 25–33.

Richardson, Henry S., and Cho, Mildred K. 2012 "Secondary Researchers' Duties to Return Incidental Findings and Individual Research Results: A Partial-Entrustment Account," *Genetics in Medicine*: doi:10.1038/gim.2012.12.

Ruger, Jennifer Prah. 2010. *Health and Social Justice* (New York: Oxford University Press).

Scanlon, T. M. 1998. *What We Owe to Each Other* (Cambridge, Mass.: Harvard University Press).

Schapiro, Tamar. 1999. "What Is a Child?" *Ethics* 109: 715–738.

Shaffer, D. N.; Yebei, V. N.; Sidle, J. E.; et al. 2006. "Equitable Treatment for HIV/AIDS Clinical Trial Participants: A Focus Group Study of Patients, Clinician Researchers, and Administrators in Western Kenya," *Journal of Medical Ethics* 32: 55–60.

Shapiro, K., and Benatar, S. R. 2005. "HIV Prevention Research and Global Inequality: Steps Towards Improved Standards of Care," *Journal of Medical Ethics* 31: 39–47.

Scheffler, Samuel. 2001. *Boundaries and Allegiances: Problems of Justice and Responsibility in Liberal Thought* (Oxford: Oxford University Press).

Shiffrin, Seana Valentine. 2008. "Promising, Intimate Relationships, and Conventionalism," *Philosophical Review* 117: 481–524.

Simmons, A. John. 2005. "The Duty to Obey and Our Natural Moral Duties," in Christopher Heath Wellman and A. John Simmons, *Is There a Duty to Obey the Law?* (Cambridge, England: Cambridge University Press): 93–189.

Sreenivasan, Gopal. 2003. "Does Informed Consent to Research Require Comprehension?" *Lancet* 362: 2016–2018.

Sreenivasan, Gopal. 2010. "Duties and Their Direction," *Ethics* 120: 465–494.

Treatment Action Campaign (TAC). 2008. *Summary of HIV Statistics for South Africa*. Available at: http://www.tac.org.za/community/keystatistics (accessed 8/21/10).

Tucker, T., and Slack, C. 2004. "Not If but How? Caring for HIV-1 Vaccine Trial Participants in South Africa," *Lancet* 362: 995.

UN General Assembly. 2008. "The Right of Everyone to the Enjoyment of the Highest Attainable Standard of Physical and Mental Health: Report of the Special Rapporteur, Paul Hunt." U.N. General Assembly, 63rd Session, Agenda Item 67(b), 11 August 2008. U.N. Doc. A/63/263. Available: http://www.essex.ac.uk/human_rights_centre/research/rth/docs/GA2008.pdf (accessed 1/16/2011).

VanDeVeer, Donald. 1986. *Paternalistic Intervention: The Moral Bounds of Benevolence* (Princeton, N.J.: Princeton University Press).

Varmus, Harold, and Satcher, David. 1997. "Ethical Complexities of Conducting Research in Developing Countries," *New England Journal of Medicine* 337: 1003–1005.

Wasswa, Henry. 2010. "Ugandan Hospitals Ration AIDS Treatment as Antiretrovirals Start to Run Out," *BMJ* 341: c3900, doi:10.1136/bmj.c3900.

Wenar, Leif. 2007. "Responsibility and Severe Poverty," in Thomas Pogge, ed., *Freedom from Poverty as a Human Right* (Oxford: Oxford University Press): 255–274.

Wenar, Leif. 2008. "Property Rights and the Resource Curse," *Philosophy & Public Affairs* 36: 2–32.

Wendler, David; Emanuel, Ezekiel J.; and Lie, Reidar K. 2004. "The Standard of Care Debate: Can Research in Developing Countries Be Both Ethical and Responsive to Those Countries' Health Needs?" *American Journal of Public Health* 94: 923–928.

Wertheimer, Alan. 2003. *Consent to Sexual Relations* (Cambridge: Cambridge University Press).

Wertheimer, Alan. 2011. *Rethinking the Ethics of Clinical Research: Widening the Lens* (Oxford: Oxford University Press).

Wertheimer, Alan, and Miller, Franklin G. 2007. "Facing Up to Paternalism in Research Ethics" *Hastings Center Report* 37 (3): 24–34.

WHO (World Health Organization). 2004. Guidance on Ethics and Equitable Access to HIV Treatment and Care, available at http://www.who.int/ethics/en/ethics_equity_HIV_e.pdf (accessed 8/21/2010).

WHO/UNAIDS. 2004. "Report from a WHO/UNAIDS Consultation, Geneva 17th-18th July 2003: Treating People with Intercurrent Infection in HIV Prevention Trials," *AIDS* 18: W1–W4.

Wolf, Susan M.; Lawrenz, Frances P.; Nelson, Charles A., Kahn, Jeffrey P., et al. 2008. "Managing Incidental Findings in Human Subjects Research: Analysis and Recommendations," *Journal of Law, Medicine, and Ethics* 36: 219–248.

World Medical Association. 2008. *Declaration of Helsinki: Ethical Principles for Medical Research Involving Human Subjects.* Revision adopted by the 52nd World Medical Assembly. Available: http://www.wma.net/en/30publications/10policies/b3/index.html (accessed 7/4/2010).

Zwitter, M., et al. 1999. "Professional and Public Attitudes towards Unsolicited Medical Intervention," *BMJ* 318: 251–253.

# INDEX

diagnoses, unexpected. *See* ancillary
care, needs, not known to
the subject *ex ante*
diarrhea, cryptosporidial, 144, 156,
171
Dickert, Neal, 20–1, 51–7
distributive objection. *See*
burdening-the-helper
objection
Doctors Without Borders, 191, 222
drug trials. *See* medical research
studies, drug trials
duties, directed. *See* obligations,
special, directed

Emanuel, Ezekiel J., 88n., 119,
121–2, 206–8, 215, 222
engagement
as a strength factor in the partial-
entrustment model, 42,
161–3
gradations in 162, 166–7,
188–9
glossed, 48–9
no longer appealed to in the
partial-entrustment model's
account of scope, 36
protocol as the basis for
assessing depth thereof,
162
entanglements, moral, xiii, 36n., 228
contrasted with promises, 210
neither associative nor voluntarily
undertaken, 209
privacy-based, 65–106,
189–190, 204
unintended obligations, by
definition, 65, 142,
209–10, 212

yet not entirely unforeseeable,
220–1
entrustment. *See also* Partial-
entrustment model of
medical researchers'
special ancillary-care
obligations
of aspects of health, 36, 38–40
Ethiopia, 144, 216
exploitation, 2, 32, 45, 108–9,
116–9, 206, 222

Food and Drug Administration
(U.S.), 178

Gates Foundation, the Bill and
Melinda, 25, 201
Gelsinger, Jesse, case of, 115
Georgetown workshop on ancillary
care (2006), xviii, 27,
178n., 200n., 216–23,
226–8
gingivitis. *See* periodontal disease
Goodin, Robert E., 14, 47n.,
99–102
Grady, Christine, 27n., 124–6,
206–8, 215, 217n., 222
gratitude
a potential ground of special
ancillary-care obligations,
12–3
as a strength factor on the
partial-entrustment
model, 42
no longer appealed to in the
partial-entrustment model's
account of scope, 36n.
*Grimes v. the Kennedy Krieger
Institute*, 180–1

right to refuse medical treatment, affirmed, 135

rights
alienation of, 87–8
basic, 111n., 112–3

risks, of study participation and otherwise, 123, 125

road accident sequelae, 40

role obligations of medical researchers. *See* ancillary care, obligations, special; medical researchers, role obligations of

Scanlon, T. M., 43

schistosomiasis, 4, 11, 16–7, 36, 49n., 50, 64, 88n., 96, 105, 174, 197, 220–1

scientific objectives. *See* medical research involving human subjects, social value thereof; medical research studies, scientific aims of

screening of potential subjects. *See* medical research subjects, borderline instances of

Shiffrin, Seana, 210

Simmons, A. John, 66

Singer, Peter A., 108–9, 118, 129, 132, 144

skin conditions, 21, 76–7

South Africa, Republic of, 7, 177, 199

special ancillary-care obligation, the, 14–5, chap. 2 *passim*, chap. 3 *passim*. *See also* ancillary care, obligations, special; partial-entrustment model of the special ancillary-care obligation

as arising from voluntary actions, 212
hunting for ancillary-care needs not required by, 182
impartiality doubly departed from by, 16–7, 19, 104–5, 126, 176, 179
justice not an apt ground for, 110–18, 208
not essentially a professional obligation, 63, 183, 198, 214–5
principal focus of this work, 2, 14, 110, 117
supplementing general grounds for ancillary-care obligation, sometimes, 20, 31, 76, 168, 204, 218–9
sometimes not, 21

sponsors of medical research studies. *See* medical research studies, sponsors thereof

spousal abuse, issue of ancillary care for, 197

stratification. *See* medical research studies, stratified

studies, medical research. *See* medical research studies

study-related care, vagueness of the notion of, 28–9

subjects of medical research. *See* medical research subjects

Sudan, 191–2, 222